Jeffrey's Journey

Healing a Child's Violent Rages

By
Debbie Jeffries
LaRayne Jeffries

with

Patricia A.S. Hernandez

Copyright 2005 Debbie Jeffries, LaRayne Jeffries
IBSN: 0-932551-66-1

Cover Design: Doubleu-gee
Cover Photography: Christian Peacock
Interior Design: Small World Productions, San Francisco
Writing Consultant: Patricia A.S. Hernandez
Strategic Advisor: Ani Chamichian
Project Editor: S. Newhart

Published by Quick American
A division of Quick Trading Company
Oakland, California

Printed in the U.S.

Jeffries, Debbie.
Jeffrey's journey : healing a child's violent rages / by Debbie Jeffries, LaRayne Jeffries with
Patricia A.S. Hernandez.
p. cm.
ISBN 0-932551-66-1

1. Obsessive-compulsive disorder in children--Alternative treatment. 2. Oppositional defiant
disorder in children--Alternative treatment. 3. Attention-deficit hyperactivity disorder—
Alternative treatment. 4. Marijuana--Therapeutic use. 5. Marijuana--Government policy--
United States. 6. Parenting.
I. Jeffries, LaRayne. II. Hernandez, Patricia A. S.
III. Title.

RJ506.O25J44 2005   618.92'85227
                                     QBI04-700549

www.quickamerican.com

Although the world is full of suffering, it is also full of the overcoming of it.

—Helen Keller

Authors' Note

Jeffrey's Journey was originally written by LaRayne Jeffries (grandmother) to document Jeffrey's younger years for the purpose of someday sharing it with him as a gift of love. As his treatment proceeded, it became obvious that this information needed to be shared with a much broader audience, specifically with other desperate parents who had out-of-control children. Debbie and LaRayne Jeffries (mother and grandmother), with the assistance of Patricia Hernandez, edited and revised the book to reflect the journey from a mother's point of view.

This book is not intended to be used as a substitute for the recommendation and supervision of a medical professional, nor do we advocate breaking the law. This story is solely offered as information on how and why my child was treated with medical marijuana.

Medical marijuana may or may not be applicable for the treatment of any or all forms of mental illness or behavior problems. It is not the purpose of this book to claim that medical marijuana will cure any illness. It can, perhaps, be one step in treatment.

Never start any treatment without first discussing it with your doctor. Medical marijuana should only be administered under the recommendation and supervision of a medical professional.

—Debbie Jeffries
—LaRayne Jeffries

Acknowledgments

First and foremost, this work of love is dedicated to my precious son, Jeffrey. His special needs have been paramount in our lives since he was born. Our hope is that through all the treatments and therapies, Jeffrey will be able to conquer what it takes to live happily and successfully in society.

Next, my eternal gratitude goes to my parents Ken and LaRayne for their untiring support and assistance throughout these years of struggle. Also, my thanks to Marge and Charlie, Jeffrey's paternal grandparents, who have been vital in the provision of necessary treatment for Jeffrey's recovery.

Valerie Leveroni Corral, and Dr. Mike Alcalay have been instrumental in Jeffrey's journey back to health. In addition, three organizations have been invaluable: Wo/Men's Alliance for Medical Marijuana (WAMM), the National Organization for the Reform of Marijuana Laws, California Chapter (NORML) and The Lindesmith Center-Drug Policy Foundation (now known as the Drug Policy Alliance [DPA]). If it had not been for their support, there is no way I could have been able to afford, financially or emotionally, to see if this treatment would help my son.

My gratitude goes to my attorney, Wendell Peters, who accepted the challenge of our controversial case. His legal guidance, expertise and support were a comfort throughout the proceedings.

I am thankful to Peter A. Clark, SJ, PhD, who graciously contributed an essay to this book. His support and expertise have been of great consolation to me.

My gratitude also goes to my two friends, Brenda Palm-Daughters and Carlene Rhondeau, who helped me through a couple of very difficult years with Jeffrey. And my friends Kendra, Christine, Sharon,

Debbie, Elizabeth, Katie, and Lindsay who I worked with at Fidelity Title were invaluable in their support.

Jeffrey's school, counselors, social workers, the County Office of Education and the County Mental Health Department have all been active in this endeavor. It has not always been smooth but they have helped with many of the rough edges.

It has been hard, it has been slow and it has been frustrating. But it has been worth it and I would do it again in a heartbeat.

May the struggles we have gone through encourage us all to "keep on keeping on" with our special needs children.

Love your guts!! xoxox

Chapter 1

I WAS SO YOUNG, AND Jeffrey was so tiny the first time I held him. Born nine weeks premature, he spent his first eleven days in the ICU and weighed a mere four pounds. The pregnancy had been difficult; I was thought to be carrying twins, but the doctors believed I'd lost one child just after the first trimester. I was also hospitalized several times because of potentially dangerous health conditions. As a newborn, Jeff was fragile, but I could already see the disposition of a fighter. All I felt was unbridled love for my little boy.

I had always dreamed of being a wife and mother, though I admit I hadn't expected it so early in life. After a childhood spent in Colorado, Alabama, Washington State, and California, my dream had been to work in the medical profession. I initially planned to enroll in a college pre-med program, and I even earned a scholarship while working as a hospital intern. After poring over what the program would entail, though, I became intimidated by the intense study load and decided it was more practical to enroll in cosmetology school, where I got my license. I worked for two years in a salon, and then, as most young people do, I decided to try a different career route. At the age of 20 I enlisted in the U.S. Navy, hoping to pursue a career in the medical field. I met Jeffrey's father, Scott, a handsome young sailor, while we were both in boot camp. Very soon, we were married. Within weeks of our nuptials, I became pregnant and was honorably discharged. When Jeff was two months old, Scott was transferred to a base in Washington State.

From the beginning, our marriage was rocky at best. Because we'd only spent a short time together before getting married, I hadn't yet seen the real man. Scott had been honest with me about his previous problems with alcohol, but he also claimed he'd been successfully treated. I soon learned otherwise—he started drinking again within months of our marriage. My new husband had neglected to tell me that he also had a drug problem; I didn't know he had been through several drug treatment programs before I'd met him. When we married, I was very naïve—Scott was a Navy man—it never even occurred to me that he would be abusing drugs. I knew that he suffered from kidney stones, and that he'd been given pain pills, but it soon became apparent that he was addicted to them. His pill bottles would go from three-quarters full to half-full overnight—he was taking many more than were prescribed. His mood swings were frighteningly erratic, and he would become fixated on otherwise mundane situations and activities.

By the time Jeff was born, Scott had revealed a very controlling and rigid personality lurking beneath his substance abuse problems. He was obsessive-compulsive to an extreme, and the drugs he was taking seemed to amplify that. For instance, we both did the chores, but Scott was always compelled to redo what I had just finished because it was never done to his impossibly high expectations. At one point, he glued the rug in front of the kitchen sink to the floor so that it would stay "perfectly" in place. He would actually use a tape measure to adjust hand towels so they would hang at exactly the same length, with exactly the same number of inches between them. The refrigerator had to be organized by both the color and height of its contents; dirty laundry had to be separated immediately, and I couldn't mop the floor—I had to clean it on my hands and knees.

The idyllic picture of motherhood I had always imagined quickly evaporated soon after we brought Jeff home. As a preemie, he faced many physical challenges during his first few months; he consistently weighed and measured far below normal for his age. From birth, he was almost impossibly active. Despite his extreme energy level, he required very little sleep at all. It was always a struggle to get Jeffrey to bed, and he seldom slept through the night. Before he was even a year old, he had learned to crawl out of his crib—we put him in a regular twin bed because we were afraid he would fall and injure himself. I had a monitor in both his room and ours, so I could hear everything. What I heard was constant motion.

Jeff remained underweight through his first year, and was completely disinterested in eating. He just didn't seem to enjoy it at all. By nine months, the military doctors on base were becoming concerned about his eating and sleeping problems and labeled him as "failing to thrive." The words alone frightened me. The doctors put him on PediaSure, a high-calorie drink meant to help maintain his weight. Despite his physical setbacks, Jeff progressed quickly intellectually and fundamentally—he talked, sat, crawled, and walked at a very young age.

Three months shy of his first birthday, he began to exhibit extreme temper tantrums. They were noticeably different from a "normal" tantrum, and Jeff's pediatrician was alarmed when he actually witnessed one of Jeff's sudden, explosive outbursts. Jeffrey was grossly aggressive with an anger like spontaneous combustion. The tantrums were not a reaction to the predictable causes—a dirty diaper, being hungry, or wanting a toy. His anger would rise to a fever pitch merely because he wasn't "moving fast enough," or his food wasn't on his high chair right away, or the milk didn't come out of his sippy-cup quickly enough.

During the daytime, if he wasn't held tightly, or rocked vigorously enough; if he wasn't bouncing in his Johnny Jump Up, or swinging in his baby swing, he would become red in the face and would cry unceasingly. When he was in his car seat, whether strapped into the car or taken out and hand-carried, he wanted the seat to be in constant rapid motion. Until he was three, the only way to get him to sleep was for me to place him in my lap, my arms crisscrossed over his chest and hands holding his thighs, rocking back and forth in an unnaturally rapid manner. This insistence on movement carried over to sleeptime, too. Even with his eyes closed, apparently asleep, he moved constantly, using every inch of his bed, rolling and crawling almost in circles.

Jeffrey's emerging personality began to echo some of Scott's odd behaviors. Jeff became obsessive about a number of things—if he didn't think there were enough "J's" or "B's" in his alphabet soup, he would fly into a rage, tossing his bowl of soup across the room. When his bed wasn't completely straight, with all seams, edges, and corners perfectly aligned, he would scream and tear the bed apart.

Life at our house on the base grew even more difficult as Jeff became more mobile. He never demonstrated any fear at all. Our first apartment had two levels, which was an accident waiting to happen. Jeff had just celebrated his first birthday when he spontaneously jumped from the top landing of the stairs. Shocked but unhurt, he laughed in delight. We were accustomed to watching him every second anyway, but now we were afraid that he would try the "funny trick" again. We moved into a single story home nearby.

On a typical day, after Scott left for work, I'd fix Jeff a bottle and we'd watch Elmo videos together, which really made him laugh. When Jeff wasn't upset, he had an infectious laugh that charmed everyone around. Often, though, his giggles were eclipsed by frustration, putting a quick end to some momentary pleasure. When

Jeff started to get restless, I'd put him in his stroller and we would take our dogs on a mile-long walk down to the seashore, which was magnificent. The stretch of beach near Whidbey Island Naval Air Base was one of the saving graces of my life back then, a place where I could realize some much needed peace. Just managing Jeff took up most of the day, and there were chores to do. I always tried hard to make sure that everything was just so when Scott arrived home—it made for an easier night. As his addiction grew, so did his verbal abuse. Scott had high highs and very low lows, and he could be mean.

We had a few friends on base—other military families—but we didn't socialize often. With the tense relationship between Scott and I, and Jeffrey's unpredictable behavior, it was usually easier just to be alone. We seldom used babysitters, which made it difficult to get out more and participate in our church and community. When Jeff was eighteen months old, we arranged to leave him with friends once a week while we volunteered as youth leaders at our church. It was clear that Jeff was becoming more and more of a burden to them, though. He was so active, and demanded so much constant attention, they were physically and mentally exhausted by the time we came to pick him up.

Sunday school at church seemed like a good way to introduce Jeff to other children in a structured environment. But being with a group of children under the supervision of several adults didn't seem to change Jeff's behavior for the better. Worse still, he began his career as an escape artist. Just after Jeff turned two, Scott and I were sitting in church listening to the sermon. Suddenly there was a commotion and the doors at the back of the church opened. The nursery attendant stepped in looking bewildered, and we all turned around to see what was going on. The attendant looked right at us. I jumped up and walked toward him. Just then, we heard the sound of a honking horn. It was a mother's instinct, I suppose—I raced toward the sound as the attendant loped alongside me, explaining that Jeffrey had somehow gone missing. By the grace of God, the driver of the car had seen Jeffrey in time; he was standing in the middle of the road.

We were becoming known around the base as the family with the "problem child." Unfortunately, our problems didn't stop there; life at home was continuing to deteriorate. After almost two years in Washington, Scott's abusive behavior had accelerated to the point where I began to fear for my safety and the safety of my son. I made the painful decision to leave my husband and move to California to be near my parents. My folks had always been there for me, and I knew they would help me now. It was obvious that Jeffrey was way too much for a single mother to handle on her own.

Chapter 2

JEFF AND I MOVED in with my parents Ken and LaRayne in December 1995. I was very fortunate in that my parents were able to help me at a time in life when children usually move out rather than move in. Later, when we relocated to our own apartment, we always stayed close to them, as I needed their help almost constantly.

I guess when it comes to family problems, you never know how you will react until you are faced with them. We are a conservative Christian family, and we rely heavily on our faith. My mother says, "No one ever knows what the future will hold. We only know Who holds it." As their first grandchild, my parents hoped to spend time with Jeff and to influence his life as only grandparents can. We had maintained frequent contact, so they already had an intimate knowledge of Jeffrey's behavior. They dearly loved their grandson, who possessed many positive characteristics—intelligence, a great sense of humor, charm, a loving side at times, and an athletic inclination—but they also recognized early on that he was a very troubled child. We all wished Jeffrey had been an even-tempered, carefree kid, but my parents have never had any second thoughts about their consistent involvement in our lives.

Because of Scott's alcohol and drug abuse, the divorce decree stipulated that he could only visit Jeff if he passed a drug test during the previous week. That happened only once, so Scott was not involved in Jeffrey's life from the divorce on. I believe Scott loved his son as best he could, and in his own way. He sent Jeff a birthday card on two occasions, but he never contacted him by phone.

Eventually, Scott received treatment from the Navy for his medical and psychological problems. While still in treatment for his substance abuse and mental health problems, he died from a drug overdose. I had prayed that Scott would eventually find a way to deal with his enormously destructive habits; he had been in so much danger and pain for so long. Sometimes it seems as if his death was inevitable, though. I was terribly sad, but in truth, I felt some relief for him knowing that his battle was now over. Jeff was only two years old when Scott and I separated, so I had no idea how the divorce would affect him. He was five when his father died, after having had very little contact with him. It must have had some meaning, even for someone so young. As Jeff grew older and wanted to know what happened, I told him an abridged version of the truth.

As soon as we moved to California, my parents helped me care for Jeff on an almost-daily basis. They were an integral part of his life. My father had retired from a career at IBM and had operated a home business in the high-tech computer field for years, with my mother acting as his assistant. They spent most of their time in the house, and they had a lot of flexibility in their schedule. Jeff would literally wipe me out with his constant spiral of activity, energy, manipulation, and anger. My parents were there for me and for Jeff when my own reserves of patience were running low.

Jeff knew his grandparents loved him. Grandma had a pet name for him, and he'd ask her often, "Do you want to watch TV with your special boy?" Then he'd run and grab an afghan, cover up and lay snuggled with his head in her lap. Such tender moments at the end of a tough day helped enormously. Perhaps because they were older, Jeff treated my parents with just a bit more respect than he treated me, and everyone else. They also had more tolerance for his misbehavior, maybe because they weren't with him constantly, as I was, and simply because there were two of them.

Jeff had a very special relationship with my father. Since his daddy was gone, Grandpa was Jeff's only male role model. Grandpa taught him all he needed to know about toilet training, and encouraged his interest in sports. He taught Jeff how to hit a whiffle ball, how to catch, how to shoot marbles, and how to play golf. At two years old, Jeff's hand/eye coordination was phenomenal. When Grandpa taught him how to bat, he started with a big beach ball. At first, he missed a lot, which frustrated him, but Grandpa was patient and managed to talk Jeff through the motions until he finally connected with the ball. Soon, he was hitting it nine times out of ten. If he missed a couple of balls in a row, though, he would get upset. Pretty soon, Grandpa was pitching too hard, too fast, or too easy; the sun was in his eyes; it was too hot; he was tired; everyone was laughing at him. If things didn't fit together exactly as Jeffrey had anticipated them in his own mind, there could be no fun, period. He always had to control the situation.

Jeffrey looked forward to going to the golf course with Grandpa. My dad would perch him on his lap in the golf cart and let him steer the one and a half miles there, then they'd feed the ducks with the cracked corn my dad always kept in the cart. After hitting some balls, they'd go to the clubhouse for a cherry Coke before "driving" back home again. Wrestling with Grandpa was another of Jeff's favorite things, along with "boys' night out." When my mom and I had something to do, or if Grandpa simply felt like spending some time with Jeff, they'd go for pizza, or to "Frucky Fried Chicken," as Jeff called it, where my dad would supply Jeffrey with a fistful of quarters for the arcade games.

These good times brought much needed joy into our difficult lives. The reality, though, was that even the enjoyable moments almost always ended on a sour note. Jeffrey simply could not find pleasure in anything for too long without being overwhelmed by his own powerful emotions. He would get angry about not being able to hit the ball well enough; he was convinced that he wasn't holding the club correctly; he complained that other people were bothering him—it was always something. It didn't matter how much he wanted to participate at the beginning; in no time, he'd made himself and anyone around him miserable.

Everyone at the Country Club swimming pool knew about Jeffrey and his outbursts; and although he always wanted to swim, he usually ended up hurting himself or someone else. He would argue, often with the lifeguards; he would disobey the rules; he wouldn't share the pool toys with the other children, which caused fights; and he was often simply banned from the entire pool area. Jeff's social skills were so lacking, no other children wanted to be around him. A few very kind lifeguards tried their best to be tolerant, but even these icons of patience could only be stretched so far. Jeff would convince one of them to toss him up in the air so he could make a big splash, but it was never high enough, never big enough, never far enough, never enough times. He found no satisfaction in the play, and he demonstrated no appreciation for the time he'd so generously been given. Events that most children look forward to, like swimming and playing ball, most often ended in frustration and anger for Jeffrey.

There were rules for Jeffrey at my parents' house, just as there were at home, and they were often forced to discipline him. It was certainly done in a loving way. They made sure he understood that punishments were not given because he was bad; it was because his actions were not acceptable. They loved the child, but hated the behavior!

Managing Jeffrey was always more complicated in public settings. It looked to any outsider witnessing one of his rages that Jeff just needed a good old-fashioned spanking. We would often overhear people muttering under their breath, "That child needs a good swat!" Others had the opposite reaction. Often, the most benign situations quickly turned into chaos, and we had learned that out-of-control situations always had lose–lose results. If certain behaviors were ignored, or even downplayed, things only got worse. What most people saw was a spoiled little boy who was allowed to get away with anything. The truth is, all parents face difficult questions when it comes to disciplining their children. We knew it was important to be consistent, and we only resorted to spanking, or the threat of a spanking, when his misbehavior was very serious.

One afternoon at the local WalMart, Jeffrey climbed out of the cart and, in a flash, disappeared in the clothes racks. Frantically, we looked and looked for him, until we eventually found him running down the aisles pulling clothes off their hangers and knocking over displays. He was completely out of control and totally unresponsive. Finally, after repeated instructions to stop, I grabbed him by the shirt collar, looked him in the eye and said, "You're going to get a spanking, young man!" A woman nearby overheard and interjected that she would call the police if I laid a hand on the poor child. In many situations, when we took the necessary steps to curb the behavior, there was always someone who was going to question what we were doing, threaten to escalate the situation, and perhaps even attract the police.

Jeff's explosive tantrums could be set off by anything: his shoelaces were not tied in equal-sized loops or the TV was on too loud. Often the cause was a complete mystery. For instance, one day when Jeff was just returning from school, my mom asked him how he was doing. He walked into the living room without a word and kicked the entertainment center door, breaking the hinges clear off.

Invariably in a restaurant, there would be a scene. The milkshake wasn't made correctly, the water had ice in it, the water didn't have ice in it, the food didn't look like what he'd ordered, the toast was too brown, the eggs were too soft, the hamburger bun fell apart too easily, the chicken wasn't on the bone. Once, after we were seated at a local restaurant, Jeff was given a child's menu, complete with crayons. Immediately, he flew into a rage. "I'm not going to eat kids' food! I want to choose from the other menu!" he shouted. No matter how we tried to explain that it was the same food, his voice got louder and louder in protest. He pushed the table and spilled water all over, then he jumped up and threw his chair down the aisle, barely missing a nearby table. Everyone in the restaurant turned to see what on earth was happening as Jeff screamed and cried. He could not be pacified. Finally, Grandpa picked him up and carried him to the restroom, trying mightily to hold Jeff's flailing arms and legs. They emerged a few minutes later, Jeffrey still screaming. We apologetically excused ourselves before ordering.

He never seemed to outgrow behavior that you would consider natural for a two-year old. He was absolutely insensitive to anyone or anything around him. It was the same behavior we faced at home; but out in public, it was louder and more disruptive. Every now and then I would see a report on TV about "out of control children." I watched through tears, my heart breaking for these families; I could see my son in their children. These people had an intimate knowledge of my life.

❧

I was exhausted almost all the time. Jeff slept very little, and therefore I slept very little, usually between two and three hours a night. I also learned to sleep with one eye open. While we were living in our own apartment, two very supportive friends stepped in to help, taking turns with my parents caring for Jeff and I. We referred to this method of aid as "tag-team discipline and behavior strategies." It was a way to cope when the constant struggle to contain, redirect, discipline, and/or supervise Jeffrey became too overwhelming for one person to handle. Similar to when a professional wrestler has had too much, there were times when I had to stretch out my hand for help. Sometimes, it literally took two people to subdue Jeff.

My parents were my main "tag-team" partners. They took Jeffrey so that I could take a sanity break or catch up on house cleaning, shopping or sleeping. There were times when I was forced to call my mom because I was so tired, so defeated, and so desperate that I could not go on. My will and my strength had left me. I never did, and never wanted to, act out in anger toward Jeff. I didn't want to lose control and do or say something I'd regret. When I felt I was approaching that point (and it happened often), I knew it was time to call for help. Mom would do her best to both soothe me and diffuse the situation. Occasionally, she would take Jeffrey back home with her. Jeffrey threw tantrums in front of everyone, but in the presence of my father, it seldom escalated to the point where he was a real danger to himself or others. Was it love that left our hearts and souls open to such hurt and frustration? If we didn't love him so much, would it have hurt less? Would it have been easier to cope with? I don't think so.

As time passed, Jeffrey progressed in many age-appropriate ways. He remained underdeveloped, growing but alway remaining smaller than other children his age. Along with the typical hurdles of a child's development, my son's erratic behaviors and actions also continued to change and evolve; he had to be watched constantly. Jeff's unpredictability complicated our lives. Even the consequences of taking the smallest risks became paramount. I literally could not go to the bathroom without taking him with me.

When he was three years old, I decided to try to shower alone. I put him in my bedroom, got him comfortable, and started his favorite video on TV. The bath adjoined my bedroom, so my shower was just a few feet away. I figured I could probably shampoo and soap in a couple of minutes if I really hurried. By the time I turned off the water, stepped out of the shower and threw a towel around myself, Jeffrey was gone. As I jogged down the hall, calling his name, I picked up the strong smell of gasoline. There he was, in the garage with an empty plastic container in his hand. He just stared at me with a faraway look. He wasn't smiling, but he didn't look upset. As I scanned the area, I could see that he'd found the lawnmower's gas tank, and had poured its contents all around: over boxes, on the car seats, in puddles on the floor. He was standing by the dryer, where he'd emptied the last of the flammable liquid. I panicked—the gas water heater was in the garage. I grabbed Jeffrey by the arm and ran back inside the house, shivering in my towel. With one hand attached to my son, I picked up the phone and called my dad. He instructed me to call the fire department and "stay calm." I can't recall what I said to the operator—the memory is a flash. I do remember being told to stay still until the firefighters arrived. They were understanding and didn't ask too many questions, but they told me that if I had used the garage door opener, the house could have blown up.

When he was just a bit older, we were sitting on the couch watching TV one night. I needed to use the bathroom, so I left him watching TV instead of taking him with me. I left the bathroom door open and I was gone for under three minutes. When I returned, I saw that Jeffrey had taken my nail polish off my desk and poured it into the computer tower. He'd completed the destruction of my hard drive by pouring sugar on top. He didn't appear to realize what he was doing. I knew he'd never seen anyone do such a thing. Then again, he'd never seen anyone remove a door hinge and shove it into a VCR, either, but he did that, too.

I had expected my life to change when I became a parent, but Jeffrey was all consuming. He had become my entire life's focus. Nothing was accomplished that wasn't planned around Jeff and his unpredictability. This was true for my parents as well, as he spent so much time at their house. Their guest room was "Jeff's" room when he stayed over, and there was a closet that had bins of toys, dress-up clothes, games, and a big blue container that my mom called "Grandma's special toys." She and Jeff had activities that were considered "theirs," including a lot of cooking, board games (his favorite was Yahtzee), putting together puzzles, and hours upon hours spent playing the "memory game," which Jeff never, ever lost. He astounded us on many occasions with his creativity, his ability to strategize, and his quick wit. Their all-time favorite thing to do was to get up early on Saturday mornings while Grandpa was gone golfing, make sausage links and hit the neighborhood garage sales.

My mother was as concerned as I was as we watched Jeff's behavior become less manageable and more volatile, so we decided to see a military doctor covered by Jeff's insurance. Determined and stubborn, Jeff had no sense of fear. At the doctor's office, he would climb up onto the examination table, throw items, refuse to let anyone near him, yell and hit, kick and bite. If we weren't watching carefully, he would jump off the table, as if to fly. In the years that followed, I would witness more than one doctor tripping over his own feet to rush across the room and catch Jeff.

I'd never even considered putting my son on medication; he was so young, and I was hoping against hope that his behavior was associated with all of the changes he'd been through. Surely, with the right therapy, or simply with growth, he'd calm down and everything would be okay. Instead, his outbursts were increasing in both frequency and intensity. For the first time, I discussed the possibility of medication with his doctor, but he was reluctant to take that step as well, though it was clear that Jeffrey's temper and aggression had to be addressed. Jeff now had his first official diagnosis: Attention Deficit/Hyperactivity Disorder (ADHD).

Attention Deficit/Hyperactivity Disorder ADHD[1]

Attention deficit hyperactivity disorder (ADHD) is a condition defined by a high level of hyperactivity combined with a lack of concentration. It is the most common behavior disorder diagnosed in children and teens. Symptoms begin in early childhood and can continue into adulthood, causing difficulties at home, school, work, and within the community if not recognized and treated.

The three groups of ADHD symptoms are inattention, impulsiveness, and hyperactivity.

We found ourselves at an impasse and decided to take a wait and see approach. For now, the available medications were not even meant for children his age.

---

1 WebMd.com. © 1995-2004 Healthwise, Incorporated; Boise, Idaho.

Chapter 3

A FTER I STARTED WORKING for a large department store as a Lancôme makeup artist, finding a place for Jeffrey to go during the day became an obvious necessity. At first, my parents babysat while I worked, but this clearly exhausted them. I needed to earn a living, and my parents simply weren't capable of caring for him all day, every day. I hated to have to depend on them so much. We knew we had to begin exposing him to other children and authority figures so that preschool and eventually kindergarten would be possible given his temperament. The search for a daycare facility began when Jeff was two. Cost was always a consideration, but safety was more important.

It wasn't terribly difficult to find a daycare that was qualified to accept a "hyperactive" little boy, but as the behavior problems increased, it became harder to find a facility that would keep him. I was always honest with the staff—Jeffrey was a handful—and I wouldn't start him anywhere if they didn't feel they could handle his constant need for supervision. Open lines of communication were always established, but I didn't go into detail about his problems; I wanted them to form their own opinions about Jeffrey.

At Jeff's very first daycare, the problems began within two weeks, and I quickly realized the impact that his behavior would have on my work schedule. My employer recognized that I had a tough situation. Still, there was a job to be done, and it certainly wasn't my employer's problem when I had emergencies, doctor's appointments, meetings, or any of the myriad of excuses that kept me from getting to work. I worked retail hours, not the usual nine-to-five, usually on weekends, evenings, and holidays—hours that daycare centers typically don't provide service. Although my employer did not have legal grounds for dismissing me due to my circumstances, the multiple absences certainly didn't help, and I understood the frustration they caused my managers and co-workers.

When I was informed that Jeffrey would have to leave daycare due to his aggression toward the other children, we found another, and then another, and then another. Jeffrey's reputation got around pretty quickly, and as soon as I would find a facility (and later, a preschool), it wouldn't be long before I was informed that he was not welcome there due to his out-of-control and non-compliant words and behavior.

We tried very hard to maintain as regular a schedule as possible. On a typical day, I'd drop Jeffrey off at either my parents' house or at daycare on my way to work, depending on my hours. At the end of the day, I would pick him up on my way home, or I'd let him sleep over at my folks' and I'd pick him up in the morning. We almost always ate dinner together, but mealtime was when problems were likely to escalate, usually ending up in a big blow-up due to Jeff's strange likes and dislikes. Seemingly little things, like having too much or too little milk in his glass, would infuriate him. If one food touched another food on his plate, he would become irate and refuse to eat. Cutting up his food was only acceptable if it was his own idea. If he asked, it was fine, but if someone else made the suggestion, he would blow: "I can do it myself! I don't need anyone else to cut it! You think I'm stupid!" He would work himself into such a state, he'd knock his plate over, crying uncontrollably. If his toast was too dark, had too many crumbs, or the butter wasn't melted properly, he would react violently. If his sandwich wasn't cut exactly corner to corner, or the squares weren't even, he would lose all composure. On Saturday mornings Jeffrey always wanted link sausages before he and Grandma headed off to the garage sales. Those special Saturday mornings could quickly turn ugly if the sausage wasn't just the right shade of brown, or if the skin on the sausage split during cooking.

Getting ready in the morning was a Keystone Cops movie without the comedy. When I was with my parents, they could entertain Jeffrey while I bathed and dressed, but when I was with him on my own, it was nearly impossible. Even as a toddler, Jeff was compulsive about his clothing and his hair, which added unavailable minutes to our preparations. He wanted different clothing than we had picked out; he wanted to change his clothes over and over again because he was never happy with how things "felt"; he insisted on combing his own hair. Once we made it to daycare, he always wanted "one more hug" before he'd let us go. One more hug always turned into 100 more hugs.

With his grandparents, Jeff was not in competition with anything or anyone for time and attention. With me, a single mom who had to get ready for work in the morning, it was very difficult. He could not understand why mommy had to go away—why I had to leave and send him to daycare or to his grandparents' house when he wanted to spend time with me, or why I had to make dinner when he wanted to play. It was as if Jeffrey was battling the world for my time. His anger was fueled by the fact that he wasn't in control.

When he spent the weekend at my parents, they could see the change in him by Sunday night—he wanted his mommy to come back. He would talk endlessly about me, waiting for me to come through the door. When I did, it was a Hallmark moment—temporarily. He'd hear my footsteps approaching and run for the door, arms extended for a hug. Then he'd stop in his tracks as if he'd seen an imaginary red flag pulled out of my purse and waved in front of him. Instantly, he was an enraged, charging bull. On other nights, he wouldn't even acknowledge me, or he'd immediately find something to argue about: "What took you so long? Why didn't you bring my skates? Why didn't you bring the dog with you?" he'd demand. He did control most every situation. And it hurt.

Although I knew Jeffrey loved me—and loves me now—most times he simply wasn't capable of treating me like he did. At night, we'd wrap up and cuddle, reading and watching TV together. It was always a struggle to keep him out of my bed at night—he routinely wanted to sneak in and curl up next to me. Despite all his anger, he was still a little boy who wanted to be held and protected. The only emotions Jeff exhibited extemporaneously were anger, rage, frustration, impatience, and intolerance. Showing positive emotion was not something Jeffrey could comprehend. Often immediately following misbehavior, he would beg to be held and loved. There were times when it took forced affection to comply with this need—he required the love, but my own hurt was so big.

The problems Jeff exhibited at home were almost always a result of his need to control and argue a point—and the only valid point was his own. He would argue until he was blue in the face about anything and everything, and would not allow anyone to tell him how to do anything. He simply had to have the last word, even if it got him in trouble—even if he was already in trouble. He was the spitting image of his father. His arguing most often took the form of sassy, disrespectful backtalk, though there were some amusing exceptions that exemplified his charming sense of humor.

We took a trip to the Pumpkin Patch when Jeff was three. As we drove along, he was perched up in his car seat, watching the farm animals as we drove along. Suddenly, he gasped: "God!" he said. We knew he had picked up some new words at daycare, but we thought we'd heard him wrong. Then, again, "God!"

"Jeffrey," I said. "We don't use God's name unless we are talking to Him or about Him, like when we say our prayers. Remember?"

"Kids at school do," he answered.

"Well, maybe they don't know how special God's name is," I tried to explain.

"But everybody else does!" he insisted.

"Jeffrey, that doesn't make it right. Please don't say God unless you are praying, okay?" I turned around and looked sternly at him.

We drove along for a few minutes in silence, and then in the rearview mirror I saw him grin. "Oh God! Look at that horse!" We laughed for ten minutes. We couldn't help it.

Every night without fail, whether at our house or at my parent's house, Jeffrey said his prayers. We always started off, "Now I lay me down to sleep..." and Jeff would continue on from there. He had a long list of people he prayed for, some of whom weren't even in his daily life anymore. His prayers were touching, and there was always a request that God would help him with his anger. When Jeff was three, he and my mom were out shopping when they came across an unfortunate looking woman. Jeffrey turned around, visibly alarmed: "Grandma, she looks like a witch!" he cried out. Mom was horrified, hoping the poor woman hadn't overheard. Later, we all had a discussion about hurting people's feelings. That night, at the end of his prayers, he added, "And God bless the woman who looks like a witch." On another night, when he was older and I had remarried, he prayed that his new brother would get a job at the skate park. After his prayers were concluded, he asked, "Grandma, if Mark gets a job at the skate park, do you think I could get free sodas?" Mom said, "Jeffrey, I didn't know Mark was even looking for a job!"

21

Jeff replied very nonchalantly, "Oh, he isn't. I just thought I would give God a good idea." All things considered, it really came as no surprise that Jeffrey would consider giving God a suggestion.

~&~

My parents and I weren't the only ones drained by Jeff's behavior; everyone around him experienced the nearly impossible burden of spending time with an uncontrollable child. The fact that at any moment, for any reason, the situation could turn upside down compounded that exhaustion; we were always on guard, waiting for the inevitable. My parents were being called upon more days than not to go pick Jeffrey up because of his misbehavior. At daycare, either Jeffrey would hurt himself through an impulsive act (jumping off a slide and biting through his tongue, or climbing on the toilet to try to get to a cupboard), or he'd hurt someone else. Each time the phone rang, we'd collectively hold our breath. On numerous occasions, he was asked to leave permanently because he was deemed to be a threat to the other children; the facility could not legally put itself in a position where he might seriously injure another child.

Jeff's exposure to other children had never been good. He couldn't spend more than a few minutes with another child without a problem arising. He always wanted to play with the neighborhood children, but he had been summarily banned from every home on the block. Jeffrey was so rowdy, rough, argumentative, and disrespectful, no one wanted him in their presence. He could never just play; it always had to be a contest of some sort. Jeffrey perceived himself as the biggest, baddest, meanest, smartest, and most talented at everything he did.

Usually he lashed out physically; he could not take "no" for an answer; he was always right; nothing was ever fair, and he was convinced that everyone was teasing him. The more children there were in any given situation, the worse his behavior was. On the playground, Jeff would crowd his way up the ladder of the slide and take his turn, even if it meant hurting other children who were in the way. He was small, but very strong. Combine that co-ordination and strength with a violent explosive personality, and he was the object of teasing, and then fear, amongst his peers at school. There was never another child who Jeff feared taking on, even if they were bigger or older. No one was exempt from Jeffrey's temper—he exhibited an extreme lack of respect for authority, and he was aggressive and hostile toward teachers as well. He hit, bit, threw things, screamed for no apparent reason, and did not follow directions.

One of the most blatant triggers for an episode was to stop an activity before it was Jeffrey's turn. It didn't matter if it was batting balls, throwing a frisbee, swinging at the park, or eating potato chips—Jeffrey had to be the one who took the last swing, threw the last ball, or ate the last chip. If he was denied his turn, no one was going to miss hearing about it. At one preschool he attended briefly, the teacher stopped batting practice just as it was Jeffrey's turn. At first, he argued that the play would continue until after his turn. Then he fussed and screamed until he became so agi-tated, he walked over to the sandbox, picked up a plastic shovel, and stormed over to the teacher. She bent down to establish eye contact with him and was stunned when Jeff hit her directly in the face with the shovel. Although it hurt, no permanent physical damage was inflicted. Particularly because of his lack of remorse, the school suspended him for several days. We were horrified.

Jeff put himself directly in the path of danger on a daily basis. He had to be watched every second because he would scale the fence and disappear in a flash, whether it was to chase down a ball or a shoe he had thrown over the fence (an especially common occurrence), or because he wanted to go home. Not only were the multiple preschools he attended concerned about the safety of the other children, they were also cautious about their own liability if he did indeed escape unnoticed.

I believe that Jeffrey knew he had problems with his emotions. He couldn't grasp it fully, but he knew he was different. For years after he was banned from a certain school, whenever we passed the school building, he'd say, "I used to go to school there, but I had to leave because I was bad." He just didn't know how to change.

Chapter 4

WHEN JEFF WAS THREE, the teachers at the preschool he was attending suggested that he might benefit from medication, namely Ritalin. They told me that they had seen children overcome some of the severe behavioral problems he was exhibiting by taking this drug. It was not a condition for his continuing attendance there. With or without medication, they had decided that they could not keep him at the school any longer, as he presented a threat to the other children. I wasn't angry—I understood.

Jeff was referred by the military base pediatrician to a private behavioral health center to be seen by a psychiatrist. Taking Jeffrey to see the doctor was a monumental feat. He was uncooperative, defiant, and he had attacked several doctors by hitting, throwing things, spitting, yelling, swearing, or kicking at them. I always needed support with me—either my mother or father (or both) accompanied us to all appointments. This doctor visit was no different. Between our own reports, those of the preschool, and the notes the pediatrician had made, including his diagnosis of ADHD, the decision to put Jeff on Ritalin seemed obvious to this psychiatrist. His notes that day observed that Jeffrey was, "aggressive, rowdy, occasionally violent and destructive, with good hearing."

Ritalin is not recommended for children under age six, and the doctor was up front in admitting that he had never prescribed Ritalin for a three year old; but he felt the situation called for "extraordinary intervention." They would "try it to see," the doctor said. Who were we to disagree with his expertise? We had already been "trying to see" if Jeff would get better, but now the problems had been confirmed and even compounded by Jeffrey's behavior in preschool. It was clearly time to explore other options. Jeff began taking Ritalin on December 23, 1996.

Ritalin [1]

Other brand names: Concerta, Metadate, Methylin

Generic name: Methylphenidate hydrochloride

Indications: Ritalin contains a mild central nervous system stimulant used in the treatment of attention deficit hyperactivity disorder (ADHD) in children. It is occasionally used in adults to treat narcolepsy.

Warnings: Excessive doses of this drug over a long period of time can produce addiction. It is also possible to develop tolerance to the drug, so that larger doses are needed to produce the original effect. Because of these dangers, be sure to check with your doctor before making any change in dosage; and withdraw the drug only under your doctor's supervision.

This drug should not be prescribed for anyone experiencing anxiety, tension, and agitation, since the drug may aggravate these symptoms.

This medication should not be taken by anyone with the eye condition known as glaucoma, anyone who suffers from tics (repeated, involuntary twitches), or someone with a family history of Tourette's syndrome (severe and multiple tics).

This drug should not be given to children under 6 years of age; safety and effectiveness in this age group have not been established.

More common side effects may include[2]: Inability to fall or stay asleep, nervousness. These side effects can usually be controlled by reducing the dosage and omitting the drug in the afternoon or evening.

In children, loss of appetite, abdominal pain, weight loss during long-term therapy, inability to fall or stay asleep, and abnormally fast heartbeat are more common side effects.

---

1 This is an abridged description of Ritalin taken from the Physician's Desk Reference (PDR) as it appears at http://www.pdrhealth.com, the official PDR online reference site for patients and laypeople (©2003 Thomson Healthcare).

2 For all drugs, the PDR states that "side effects cannot be anticipated," and suggests that "only your doctor can determine if it is safe for you." Drug side effects are often quite lengthy. These listings are abbreviated for the sake of brevity. For more complete information, please refer to www.pdrhealth.net or other reliable medical reference sources, or ask your physician.

By January 1997, Jeff's behavior had still not improved. The psychiatrist recommended a child psychology evaluation for behavioral disorders, and continued monitoring him closely on the trial of Ritalin. In February, the staff at Jeff's new preschool reported that he seemed to be focusing better. In March, it was noted that his behavior was generally improving, but that he was still very hyperactive. The dosage of Ritalin was increased, and the doctor recommended to the county education program that Jeff needed care beyond the capability of a regular preschool facility. He also suggested therapy, behavior modification classes, further exploration into medication, and careful monitoring.

Ritalin actually seemed to exacerbate Jeff's instability, especially when the dosage was increased; but the behavior he had exhibited in front of the doctors and preschool teachers was so extreme that its continued use was deemed appropriate. Jeffrey became more agitated and active. Ritalin was like putting him at warp speed—and it was frightening because it was experimental. Even though Jeff had barely moved out of his toddler years, I began to fear for my own safety—that's how angry and aggressive he could be.

In September 1997, a second military base pediatrician, referred by the psychiatrist, noted, "Jeffrey is still having problems with violence, temper, disregarding. A little better on focusing attention. An eye tic has developed. As a diagnosis, behavioral disorder and ADHD." He recommended that Jeff see a behavioral medicine specialist. This new doctor changed his medication from Ritalin to Dexedrine, and referred him to a local child psychiatrist for follow-up. Three days later, the child psychiatrist noted that, "...he was suspended from school for having very aggressive combative behavior and explosive anger." She diagnosed him with impulse disorder (nonspecified), confirmed the ADHD, and started Jeffrey on a trial of Imipramine.

Three weeks later, his primary pediatrician noted, "he was so aggressive he could not return to school on the stimulants he was taking. He is not sleeping and has very poor attention. He is alert, very active and not cooperative." He recommended that Jeffrey return to the child psychiatrist, who on that very day added Mellaril to the Dexedrine and Imipramine to combat the defiance and aggressive hostility.

Impulse Disorder[3] (not otherwise specified)

Impulse Disorder is a failure or extreme difficulty in controlling impulses despite the negative consequences. A diagnosis of impulse disorder might include the failure to control impulses to engage in gambling, violent behavior, sexual behavior, fire starting, stealing, and self-abusive behaviors. Types of impulse specific impulse disorders include Intermittent Explosive Disorder, Kleptomania, Pathological Gambling, Pyromania and Trichotillomania

Mellaril[4] (brand name)

Generic name: Thioridazine hydrochloride

Indications: Mellaril is primarily used in the treatment of schizophrenia. Because it has been known to cause dangerous heartbeat irregularities, it is usually prescribed only when at least two other medications have failed.

Warnings: The danger of potentially fatal cardiac irregularities increases when Mellaril is combined with any medication that prolongs a part of the heartbeat known as the QTc interval. Many drugs prescribed for heartbeat irregularities prolong the QTc interval and should never be combined with Mellaril. Other drugs to avoid when taking Mellaril include Luvox, Norvir, Paxil, Pindolol, Prozac, Rescriptor, and Tagamet. Make sure the doctor knows you are taking Mellaril whenever a new drug is prescribed.

Mellaril may cause tardive dyskinesia--a condition marked by involuntary muscle spasms and twitches in the face and body.

In rare cases, Mellaril has been known to trigger blood disorders and seizures.

---

3 Taken from http://allpsych.com, the psychology online classroom.

4 This is an abridged description of Mellaril taken from the Physican's Desk Reference (PDR) as it appears at http://www.pdrhealth.com, the official PDR online reference site for patients and laypeople (©2003 Thomson Healthcare).

Common side effects[5]**:** Agitation, anemia, asthma, body spasm, breast development in males, chewing movements, confusion (especially at night), constipation, diarrhea, discolored eyes, drowsiness, dry mouth, excitement, fever, headache, intestinal blockage, involuntary movements, irregular blood pressure, pulse, and heartbeat, jaw spasm, loss of appetite, mouth puckering, muscle rigidity, nasal congestion, nausea, overactivity, painful muscle spasm, paleness, pinpoint pupils, protruding tongue, psychotic reactions, rapid heartbeat, redness of the skin, restlessness, rigid and masklike face, sensitivity to light, skin pigmentation and rash, sluggishness, strange dreams, sweating, swelling, tremors, vomiting, weight gain, yellowing of the skin and whites of eyes

Dexedrine[6] (brand name)

Generic name: Dextroamphetamine sulfate

Indications: Dexedrine is a stimulant that is prescribed to help treat narcolepsy (recurrent "sleep attacks") and Attention Deficit/Hyperactivity Disorder.

Warnings: Because it is a stimulant, this drug has high abuse potential. There is some concern that Dexedrine may stunt a child's growth. For the sake of safety, any child who takes Dexedrine should have his or her growth monitored. This drug is not recommended for children under 3 years of age.

Common side effects[7]**:** Excessive restlessness, overstimulation

Imipramine[8] (generic name)

Brand name: Tofranil

Indications: Tofranil is a tricyclic antidepressant that is used to treat depression. It may also be used to treat attention deficit/hyperactivity disorder in children, obsessive-compulsive disorder, panic disorder, bulimia, or as a short-term treatment for bedwetting in children under the age of 6.

---

5 For more complete information, please refer to www.pdrhealth.net or other reliable medical reference sources, or ask your physician.

6 This is an abridged description of Dexedrine taken from the Physician's Desk Reference (PDR) as it appears at http://www.pdrhealth.com, the official PDR online reference site for patients and laypeople (©2003 Thomson Healthcare).

7 For more complete information, please refer to www.pdrhealth.net or other reliable medical reference sources, or ask your physician.

8 This is an abridged description of Imipramine taken from the PDR as it appears at http://www.pdrhealth.com, the official PDR online reference site for patients and laypeople (©2003 Thomson Healthcare).

Warnings: Tofranil or any tricycle antidepressant may cause a serious or fatal reaction if it is taken with a MAO inhibitor.

Tofranil should only be used in children to treat bedwetting, and its use should be limited to short-term therapy. Safety and effectiveness in children under the age of 6 have not been established.

Common side effects[9]: Agitation, anxiety, congestive heart failure, constipation or diarrhea, cough, fever, sore throat, delusions, disorientation, dizziness, drowsiness, dry mouth, episodes of elation or irritability, fatigue, fever, flushing, frequent urination or difficulty or delay in urinating, hallucinations, headache, heart attack, heart failure, high blood pressure, high or low blood sugar, high pressure of fluid in the eyes, hives, inflammation of the mouth, insomnia, intestinal blockage, irregular heartbeat, lack of coordination, lightheadedness, loss of appetite, nausea, nightmares, odd taste in mouth, palpitations, purple or reddish-brown spots on skin, rapid heartbeat, restlessness, ringing in the ears, seizures, sensitivity to light, skin itching and rash, stomach upset, stroke, sweating, swelling due to fluid retention (especially in face or tongue), swollen glands, tingling, pins and needles, and numbness in hands and feet, tremors, visual problems, vomiting, weakness, weight gain or loss, yellowed skin and whites of eyes

In children, anxiety, collapse, constipation, convulsions, emotional instability, fainting nervousness, sleep disorders, stomach and intestinal problems, and tiredness are the most common side effects.

■

Now that multiple doctors were involved, it was painfully clear that each one was going to have his or her own opinion when it came to Jeffrey's treatment. Although Jeff displayed the same type of violence and anger at his various appointments, each doctor had a different take on which medications or behavioral modification therapies would benefit him most. The terms they used to describe his conditions remained consistent, and we could see that Jeffrey displayed classic symptoms of the various diagnoses. The "labels" made sense to us; we just didn't always feel comfortable with the treatment. The doctors never seemed to be overly concerned about the effects the drugs might be having, even given Jeff's size and age.

Despite the more rigorous efforts to treat him, Jeff's violence

9 For more complete information, please refer to www.pdrhealth.net or other reliable medical reference sources, or ask your physician.

was gaining momentum. He couldn't be trusted with other children, animals, or himself. His outbursts were often directed at me—throwing things, head butting, kicking and biting—and he hurt me more than once. He was very destructive and broke things—windows, screens, toys, shelves in the refrigerator, and VCR's—anything within arm's reach. Often, the items were expensive and almost impossible for me to replace with my low income. At a friend's home, Jeffrey felt he wasn't getting enough attention. He picked up a very special crystal bowl my friend's deceased husband had given her. We instructed him to put it down, but he glared at us, lifted his arm, and dropped the bowl onto the tile floor, smashing it into a million pieces. He had no remorse; it was our fault because we'd been talking. There was nothing I could do to replace my friend's priceless keepsake.

One of the most disturbing aspects of Jeffrey's behavior was his infatuation with killing—himself, me, and animals, mainly. He spoke endlessly about cutting someone's head off. His most unsettling way of acting out was to torture animals. For a time, we had a blind dog; Jeff would punch and kick him, hard, so I finally gave the dog away. Sometimes he would sneak a table knife from the kitchen and go outside to stab through the slats of the neighbor's fence, trying to hurt their dogs. Amazingly, Jeff didn't even remember these episodes, which concerned me even more. Most children do fantasize, they do talk about blood and gore, they pretend; but with Jeffrey's hair-trigger violence, you never knew what lines might be crossed.

We continued to watch for any improvement, but in most cases if there were no positive results from any given drug after six weeks, or if the medication actually made things worse, I saw no reason for my son to keep taking it. I literally had to plead with the doctors sometimes to discontinue certain medications

Our quest for help was not limited to pharmaceuticals, either. In addition to lots of prayer, we tried just about everything: we eliminated red food coloring, sugar, red meat, and preservatives; he was tested for food allergies; we tried supplements from the health food store; we sought out psychiatric care and individual therapy; we learned behavioral modification techniques; and we enrolled in parenting classes. If you can name it, we probably tried it.

When it came to discipline, my parents tried to follow my lead, which usually consisted of whatever the therapist or psychiatrist recommended as the "latest and greatest" technique for coping with Jeffrey's behavior. Naturally, every doctor had a different approach. Constantly seeking something that would promote a difference in his behavior, I gave any and everything a chance: we tried spanking—we also tried not spanking. Time-outs were useless; counting to ten yielded no results; we attempted to forcibly restrain him. We even gave ignoring the behavior a chance. Nothing worked.

We regret one psychiatrist's directions to this day. This doctor came highly recommended and specialized in pediatric/adolescent care. During an office visit with my parents and I, Jeffrey was, as usual, defiant, aggressive, and uncooperative. He climbed under a chair and refused to come out, so the doctor decided to forcibly remove him. Jeffrey continued kicking, swinging his arms, yelling, and trying to bite. The doctor explained to him that if he didn't stop, he would have to be restrained. Jeffrey ignored him, so the doctor pulled him into his lap between his knees, wrapped his legs around Jeffrey's legs, and his arms around Jeffrey's chest, and held him tightly. Jeffrey went ballistic. He yelled, swore, headbutted, and fought with every ounce of his formidable strength. The doctor continued to repeat that he would let him go if Jeff stopped fighting. Jeffrey resisted for at least ten minutes—it felt more like hours as we sat there silent, in tears.

Adderall[10] (brand name)

Generic ingredients: Amphetamines

Indications: Adderall is prescribed in the treatment of Attention Deficit Hyperactivity Disorder (ADHD) and narcolepsy (uncontrollable attacks of sleep).

Warnings: Adderall, like all amphetamines, has a high potential for abuse.

Adderall can make tics and twitches worse.

At present, there has been no experience with long-term Adderall therapy in children. However, other amphetamine-based medications have been known to stunt growth, so your doctor will need to watch the child carefully.

Common side effects[11]: Accidental injury, constipation, depression, diarrhea, dizziness, dry mouth, emotional instability, exaggerated feelings of well-being, fatigue, fever, headache, high blood pressure, hives, impotence, indigestion, infections, insomnia, loss of appetite, mental disturbances, nausea, nervousness, overstimulation, rapid or pounding heartbeat, restlessness, stomach and intestinal disturbances, tremor, twitches, unpleasant taste, vomiting, weakened heart, weight loss, worsening of tics (including Tourette's syndrome)

■

Finally, out of sheer exhaustion, Jeffrey began to calm down. After a few minutes, the doctor asked if he would sit quietly and talk. Jeffrey whimpered a sullen "yes," and the doctor released his grip. Immediately, the violence began again, and Jeff yelled, "You can't do that to me!" Once again, the doctor wrapped his arms around him for what seemed like an eternity. When he was released the second time, Jeffrey sulked and refused to speak. As if he had found the cure-all to Jeff's problems, the doctor instructed us to use this technique any time Jeff was violent. We were all gravely concerned about this particular method, but nothing we had tried previously had succeeded. He was the professional, after all. This particular doctor also prescribed Adderall.

All of the behavior modification and parenting classes I had

---

10 This is an abridged description of Adderall taken from the Physician's Desk Reference (PDR) as it appears at http://www.pdrhealth.com, the official PDR online reference site for patients and laypeople (©2003 Thomson Healthcare).

11 For more complete information, please refer to www.pdrhealth.net or other reliable medical reference sources, or ask your physician.

attended stressed that if you started something, you had to be consistent and follow through. I couldn't restrain Jeff at home or at school, and not restrain him out in public. Any time we were around other people, I discovered that there was no way to do a take-down of a five-year-old child without drawing attention.

One Sunday afternoon, Jeff and I took a trip to the grocery store—I usually tried to arrange to shop when Jeff wasn't along. The cashiers at this store knew Jeffrey well—they had seen his outbursts on many occasions. At the checkout counter, Jeffrey went into a rage—he rocked the cart, threw things, and swore. When I tried to remove him from the cart's seat, he bit into my hand, tearing a quarter-sized chunk of flesh loose. Blood gushed everywhere as my cart of groceries tipped over. The entire store gathered around to witness the display.

Finally, I was able to get him into a prone position and restrain him; it took fifteen minutes before he was quiet enough to be released. I returned him to the cart as the clerk picked up my groceries and I wrapped my bleeding hand. Trying to appear undaunted was exasperating, exhausting, and embarrassing. It was Mother's Day. The clerk looked at me and said, "Debbie, I don't know how you do it. In my book, you get the mother of the century award!" Somehow, that didn't make me feel any better. Jeff remembered nothing of the incident until years later, when he said to me, "Mom, I'll bet that didn't help when the guy told you that you won the mother of the century award, did it?"

Maybe this technique works for some; but the more Jeffrey felt restrained and boxed in, the more he fought. Jeff's sense of "coming first" was paramount, and this method was not "fair" in his opinion. We discontinued the technique after discussing it with the doctor, but the damage had already been done. Now, Jeffrey was repelled by being held, or even by being touched. He has never completely regained the physical trust he'd had prior to this experiment.

～

Finally, Jeff's behavior escalated to the point where he was banned from our county's daycare system entirely. The hammer fell one morning when I dropped Jeffrey off and continued on to work. By the time I arrived, there was already a message waiting: I had to come and get him immediately. When his teacher had disallowed him from going out the door to say goodbye to me one more time, he had grabbed a pencil and stabbed her repeatedly in the arm. My parents picked him up and kept him every day for two or three weeks while I searched for a facility who might accept him.

I was finally able to find a new preschool, and over the following months, this school went above and beyond what any facility had done before. They worked closely with us, making every conceivable effort to accommodate Jeff's problems. They also kept him enrolled much longer than I expected. This school recognized that he was a gifted child in many ways, but that his antisocial, aggressive behavior was a serious problem. His teacher wrote: "Jeff is a very bright and likable boy when he is not out of control. He does well for a while, then he reverts back to the violent and aggressive behavior. I love Jeffrey, but I'm afraid for the safety of the other children and adults when he is acting out. I have worked with him for three months on controlling his negative behavior. He responds to me usually, but these last weeks, he has been screaming at me and the other children. He will throw toys and objects down. He is hitting the teachers, too. He needs the help of a child mental health care professional. Any suggestions to me would be appreciated."

A few weeks later, Jeff worked himself into such a state of rage that he picked up a desk and upended it, warning the teacher that he was going to throw it at her. At four years old, Jeff was 32 inches tall and 36 pounds—the desk probably weighed as much as he did; but Jeff had the temperament of a Tasmanian devil. The potential for harm couldn't have been more obvious; the threat was very real. The school wasn't able to reach me or my parents for several hours, so Jeffrey was required to spend that time in the principal's office. During those few hours, she had a glimpse of what we lived through every day. Until then, she had been a very supportive force in Jeffrey's life, but she now recognized that providing a safe environment for her staff and the other students had to come first.

In the end, it was a combination of Jeff's out-of-control behavior and pressure from other parents that forced the final decision that he would have to leave the only preschool that had cared about him. By the age of five, Jeffrey had been in and out of at least eight different daycare or preschool programs. The principal of this final preschool suggested that Jeffrey be evaluated by the IEP (Individual Educational Plan) program. With the realization that there was nothing left they could do, she called for the school district to become involved and arranged for IEP testing.

Within our county's school district, a student is referred to IEP evaluation once he or she has exhibited repeated questionable behavior that could potentially prevent an education in a typical classroom setting. This consists of a lengthy series of meetings and tests for the purpose of appropriate educational placement. Follow-up meetings are scheduled on a mandatory basis, at least twice a year. Students are reevaluated every third year.

The IEP team includes the parents, educators, support staff, and mental health practitioners. There are many components—everything from reports from teachers, psychologists, family and doctors, to extensive testing (Vineland Adaptive Behavior Scales, Development Test of Visual Motor Integration, Bender Visual Motor Gestalt Test, and Behavior Assessment System for Children), behavioral observations at home and school, and academic skills—

that make up the composite recommended placement for the student. There are also federally mandated requirements that need to be met for Severely Emotionally Disturbed (SED) students. The IEP determines whether a student has met such requirements.

Jeff's IEP testing began in November 1997, and showed very negative results. The goal was to strategize the best educational plan—to determine which school would meet his needs in the least restrictive environment; which type of classroom (Severely Emotionally Disabled, Special Day Class, or Resource Classroom, for example) was appropriate, what type of services (mental health, occupational therapy, etc.) were necessary, what transportation would be used, and how safety issues would be dealt with. The recommendation was for Jeff to attend a non-public SED (Severely Emotionally Disabled) school, which he began in May 1998. It was a county school, and transportation was to be provided. Jeff would receive age-appropriate classroom instruction, group and individual therapy, and he would be seen by a psychiatrist. We knew that if he didn't get the help he needed, Jeff would never be able to function in a normal school setting. As we soon learned, even a special needs school was ill equipped to deal with him.

Chapter 5

BY THE MIDDLE OF May in 1998, Jeff's child psychiatrist requested that he be transferred back to a behavioral medicine doctor as he had begun to display, "strange and unusual behavior with significant behavioral disorder." We saw the doctor on May 20th. Mom and I took Jeff to a large military medical facility about 80 miles from home to see this pediatric specialist. From the moment we got there, Jeff was extremely uncooperative. While he screamed, kicked and flailed his arms, we forcibly removed him from the car, taking our punches and scratches. When he refused to move from the spot, we took turns picking him up and carrying him until we got into the building. Once inside, he blew up again, throwing himself on the ground and screaming that he didn't want to see a "stupid doctor." We waited for the storm to break, but there was no changing his mind. We were exhausted by the time we reached the reception area. Jeffrey was just catching his second wind when we were asked to move to a different waiting room area. When the nurse came, he physically resisted being weighed or having his blood pressure taken. The nurse, my mom, and I were drained and soaked with perspiration.

"I won't talk to you!" Jeff screamed at the doctor, before yanking his stethoscope from around his neck and throwing it to the ground, breaking it. Soon, books were flying. I picked him up off the table and sat in a chair holding him in my lap, trying to hold him securely so that he wouldn't destroy anything else. He leaned forward as far as he could and then flung his head back with all his might, head-butting me directly in the mouth. Blood started to flow along with my tears, and my mom took him while I ran from the room. Apparently, the sight of my blood squelched his temper; for the first time in an hour, he relaxed in her arms. When I composed myself and entered the room, he ran to my side and hugged me. He wanted me to love on him. There were no "I'm sorrys," though. The doctor ordered neurological evaluation tests and took Jeffrey off of all the meds the psychiatrist had put him on. Two weeks later, he introduced Clonidine.

Clonidine (generic name Clonodine hydrochloride)[1]

Brand name: Catapres

Indications: Catapres is taken orally or worn as a transdermal patch. It is prescribed for high blood pressure. It is effective when used alone or with other high blood pressure medications. Doctors also prescribe Catapres for alcohol, nicotine, or benzodiazepine (tranquilizer) withdrawal; migraine headaches; smoking cessation programs; Tourette's syndrome (tics and uncontrollable utterances); narcotic/methadone detoxification; premenstrual tension; and diabetic diarrhea.

Warnings: Catapres should not be stopped suddenly. Headache, nervousness, agitation, tremor, confusion, and rapid rise in blood pressure can occur. If Catapres is taken with certain other drugs, the effects of either could be increased, decreased, or altered. Safety and effectiveness of the Catapres tablets and patch in children below the age of 12 have not been established.

Common side effects[2]: More common side effects may include: Agitation, constipation, dizziness, drowsiness, dry mouth, fatigue, impotence, loss of sex drive, nausea, nervousness, sedation (calm), vomiting, weakness

At the SED school, the in-house psychiatrist preferred seeing the students there exclusively, so Jeffrey's care was transferred to

---

1 This is an abridged description of Clonidine from http://www.pdrhealth.com, the official online patient resource based on PDR (Copyright ©2003 Thomson Healthcare).

2 For more complete information, see www.pdrhealth.com, another reliable medical reference source, or ask your physician.

him. During their first meeting, he reported that he had already read over Jeffrey's medical reports. His observation was that Jeffrey was "very sad, still aggressive, violent, and mean." He took Jeff off the Clonidine and instead prescribed Depakote. This drug had a very serious psychotic side effect. The night he started it, I awoke to find him standing beside my bed, his hands around my throat. He was trying to strangle me. I sat up, pulled his hands away, and asked him what he was doing. "I have robots living in my stomach," he said with an eerie calm. "They're telling me to kill my mother."

Depakote[3]

Generic name: Divalproex sodium (Valproic acid)

Indications: Depakote, in both delayed-release tablet and capsule form, is used to treat certain types of seizures and convulsions. The delayed-release tablets are also used to control the manic episodes--periods of abnormally high spirits and energy--that occur in bipolar disorder (manic depression). An extended-release form of this drug, Depakote ER, is prescribed to prevent migraine headaches.

Warnings: Depakote can cause serious or even fatal liver damage, especially during the first 6 months of treatment. Children under 2 years of age are the most vulnerable, especially if they are also taking other anticonvulsant medicines and have certain other disorders such as mental retardation. The risk of liver damage decreases with age; but you should always be alert for symptoms.

Researchers have not established the safety and effectiveness of Depakote for prevention of migraines in children or in adults over 65.

Common side effects[4]: Abdominal pain, abnormal thinking, breathing difficulty, bronchitis, bruising, constipation, depression, diarrhea, dizziness, emotional changeability, fever, flu symptoms, hair loss, headache, incoordination, indigestion, infection, insomnia, loss of appetite, memory loss, nasal inflammation, nausea, nervousness, ringing in the ears, sleepiness, sore throat, tremor, vision problems, vomiting, weakness, weight loss or gain.

---

3 This is an abridged description of Depakote from http://www.pdrhealth.com, the official online patient resource based on the PDR (Copyright ©2003 Thomson Healthcare).

4 For more complete information, see www.pdrhealth.com, another reliable medical reference source, or ask your physician.

Tenex[5]

Generic name: Guanfacine hydrochloride

Indications: Tenex is given to help control high blood pressure. This medication reduces nerve impulses to the heart and arteries; this slows the heartbeat, relaxes the blood vessels, and thus reduces blood pressure. Tenex may be given alone or in combination with other high blood pressure medications.

Warnings: Discontinuing Tenex abruptly may result in nervousness, rapid pulse, anxiety, heartbeat irregularities, and so-called rebound high blood pressure (higher than before you started taking Tenex).

The safety and effectiveness of Tenex have not been established in children under 12 years of age.

An overdose can cause lethargy, extremely low blood pressure and can have serious life threatening consequences.

Common side effects[6]**:** Constipation, dizziness, dry mouth, fatigue, headache, impotence, sleepiness, weakness

∎

Jeffrey told the psychiatrist that he couldn't sleep because of nightmares about dinosaurs and robbers. He also spoke of missing his father. The psychiatrist added Post Traumatic Stress Disorder (PTSD), Bipolar Disorder, Obsessive-Compulsive Disorder (OCD), and Tourette's Syndrome to Jeff's diagnoses. He also added Imipramine and Tenex (Guanfacine) and increased his Depakote, with the rationale that the Depakote would help him sleep better. It had the opposite effect—instead of sleeping, Jeffrey was up every night at two a.m. doing homework or washing dishes. His impulsivity, defiance, hyperactivity and explosive aggression continued, so the psychiatrist increased the Imipramine. A month or so later, Jeffrey kicked this doctor squarely in the crotch and spit in his face. His notes included the following: "Reported violence up. Jeffrey looks very tired. Only participates in group when asked a direct question."

---

5 This is an abridged description of Tenex taken from http://www.pdrhealth.com, the official online patient resource based on the PDR (Copyright ©2003 Thomson Healthcare).

6 For more complete information, see www.pdrhealth.com, another reliable medical reference source, or ask your physician.

Post Traumatic Stress Disorder (PTSD)[7]

A type of anxiety disorder that can develop after experiencing a very traumatic or life-threatening event. Post-traumatic Stress Disorder can be terrifying and even disabling for some people. It can cause flashbacks, sleep problems and nightmares, feelings of isolation, guilt, paranoia, and sometimes panic attacks. Examples of traumatic events that can lead to PTSD include:

- War combat
- Terrorist attacks
- Violent crimes, such as a rape, domestic abuse, or physical assault
- A serious accident or injury
- A natural disaster, such as a fire, tornado, flood, or earthquake. Ongoing physical or sexual abuse

Common symptoms of PTSD include:

- Recurring, intrusive, and distressing memories of the event.
- Avoiding situations that remind you of the event.
- Becoming emotionally numb and withdrawing.
- Difficulty sleeping and concentrating, and fearing for your personal safety.

PTSD usually develops within three months of the trauma, although it may not develop until months or years later. Symptoms last around three months in up to half of those who get PTSD. Others may have symptoms that come and go over several years.

Bipolar Disorder (BD)[8]

Bipolar disorder (also called manic-depressive disorder) is a medical condition that causes extreme mood changes that alternate between episodes of depression and mania. One may return to a normal mood between these extremes. However, a depressive or manic episode can appear suddenly, without an obvious trigger.

The cause of bipolar disorder is not known. It may run in families. Bipolar disorder may be linked to problems in the balance of chemicals in the brain. It may also be linked to problems with how the endocrine system works. Another theory is that the structure or size of certain parts of the brain may be abnormal.

---

7 WebMd.com, © 1995-2004, Healthwise, Incorporated, P.O. Box 1989, Boise, ID 83701.

8 WebMd.com © 1995-2004, Healthwise, Incorporated, P.O. Box 1989, Boise, ID 83701.

Bipolar disorder is common and occurs equally among males and females. Over 3 million Americans—about 1% of the population—suffer from bipolar disorder, with similar rates existing in other countries. Bipolar disorder often begins between the ages of 15 and 24, although diagnosis and treatment may not begin until several years later.

Certain childhood attention disorders can mimic symptoms of bipolar disorder. Research is ongoing to determine whether a connection exists between attention-deficit hyperactivity disorder (ADHD) and bipolar disorder. Regardless, while symptoms can be similar, ADHD is a separate disorder that is very different from bipolar disorder and has different treatment. Your doctor can distinguish and properly diagnose ADHD with a normal evaluation. Although most cases of ADHD are not related to bipolar disorder, ADHD can occur along with bipolar disorder in children.

■

We were with the psychiatrist when Jeffrey exhibited the trademark manifestations of his extreme anger and aggression—biting, hitting and screaming. He was completely out of control, and the doctor declared it an emergency situation. He felt Jeff required hospitalization and said he feared for my safety if I tried to drive home with Jeff in this mental state. But putting Jeff into an in-patient hospital meant handcuffing him and transporting him in a police car. That was the rule, regardless of his age. It was absolutely out of the question in my mind. Jeffrey needed help, not more trauma, so I refused to allow it. We made it home.

The new diagnoses of Intermittent Explosive Disorder (IED) and Severe Conduct Disorder were made, and ADHD and Bipolar Syndrome were now ruled out. Risperdal was introduced. A week later, the psychiatrist's report read: "During this visit, Jeffrey continued to be hyper, demanding and violent. He bit the doctor. The episode lasted over half an hour and then suddenly, when the doctor suggested in-patient, Jeffrey became very sweet and cooperative."

Obsessive Compulsive Disorder (OCD)[9]

One of the anxiety disorders, OCD is defined by the need of the individual to always have certain parameters met. It is a potentially disabling condition that can persist throughout a person's life. The individual who suffers from OCD becomes trapped in a pattern of repetitive thoughts and behaviors that are senseless and distressing but extremely difficult to overcome. OCD occurs in a spectrum from mild to severe, but if severe and left untreated, it can destroy a person's capacity to function at work, at school, or even in the home.

Although OCD symptoms typically begin during the teenage years or early adulthood, recent research shows that some children develop the illness at earlier ages, even during the preschool years. Studies indicate that at least one-third of cases of OCD in adults began in childhood. Suffering from OCD during early stages of a child's development can cause severe problems for the child. It is important that the child receive evaluation and treatment by a knowledgeable clinician to prevent the child from missing important opportunities because of this disorder.

Tourette's Syndrome[10]

Tourette's Syndrome, also referred to as Tourette's disorder (TD), is a condition in which a person exhibits involuntary body movements (motor tics) or vocalizations that may consist of actual words or just sounds (vocal tics). This neurological disorder usually begins early in life and may range from mild or infrequent to severe and frequent in its manifestation. Motor tics often develop between the ages of 3 and 8, and vocal tics can begin as early as 3 but tend to follow the onset of motor tics by a few years. TD outbursts are commonly stereotyped as uncontrollable outbursts of cursing, obscene gestures or uncontrollable, sexually inappropriate touching. This is not true. Very few people with TD have these types of tics.

Typically, the behavioral manifestations of Tourette's are at their most severe around the age of 12, but they can continue into adulthood. The uncontrollable behaviors manifested with Tourette's may affect a child's self-esteem and relationships with friends and family, and may also interfere with his or her ability to learn.

---

9 (Obsession-Compulsive Disorder, National Institute of Mental Health, Revised 1996. Reprinted 1999. 20p. NIH 99-3755)

10 WebMd.com, © 1995-2004, Healthwise, Incorporated, P.O. Box 1989, Boise, ID 83701.

Intermittent Explosive Disorder (IED)[11]

Marked by sudden, unpredictable acts of violent, aggressive behavior in otherwise normal persons. The reaction is out of proportion to the event that triggers or provokes the outburst. The exact cause is not known. There may be a link between this disorder and mild neurological problems similar to those associated with some learning disabilities.

A person who has Intermittent Explosive Disorder fails to resist aggressive impulses that result in serious assaultive acts or destruction of property. IED is typically diagnosed when the aggressive episodes are not better accounted for by another mental disorder (e.g., Antisocial Personality Disorder, Borderline Personality Disorder, a Psychotic Disorder, a Manic Episode, Conduct Disorder, or Attention-Deficit/Hyperactivity Disorder) and are not due to the direct physiological effects of a substance (e.g., a drug of abuse, a medication) or a general medical condition (e.g., head trauma, Alzheimer's disease).

Conduct Disorder (CD)[12]

A repeated and persistent pattern of violating the basic rights of others or violating social rules. People with Conduct Disorder may:

- Harm or threaten to harm other people or animals. They may bully or threaten people, initiate physical fights, or be cruel to animals.

- Cause property damage or loss. They often may deliberately cause a fire or otherwise destroy property.

- Lie, cheat, or steal. They may break into someone's house or shoplift. They may lie to obtain things that they want or to avoid consequences.

- Violate household or social rules. Children with Conduct Disorder may stay out at night without permission from their parents. They may run away from home or be absent from school without permission.

For someone to be diagnosed as having Conduct Disorder, three or more behaviors need to have been present during the past 12 months, with at least one behavior within the past six months.

11 WebMd.com, © 1995-2004, Healthwise, Incorporated, P.O. Box 1989, Boise, ID 83701; (American Psychiatric Association. (1994). Diagnostic and statistical manual of mental disorders, fourth edition. Washington, DC: American Psychiatric Association.)

12 WebMd.com, © 1995-2004, Healthwise, Incorporated, P.O. Box 1989, Boise, ID 83701.

Risperdal[13]

Generic name: Risperidone

Indications: Risperdal is prescribed for the treatment of schizophrenia, the crippling mental disorder that causes victims to lose touch with reality. Risperdal is thought to work by muting the impact of dopamine and serotonin, two of the brain's key chemical messengers.

Warnings: Risperdal may cause tardive dyskinesia, a condition that causes involuntary muscle spasms and twitches in the face and body. This condition can become permanent.

Risperdal may mask signs and symptoms of drug overdose and of conditions such as intestinal obstruction, brain tumor, and Reye's syndrome (a dangerous neurological condition that may follow viral infections, usually occurring in children).

Risperdal can also cause difficulty when swallowing, which in turn can cause a type of pneumonia.

Risperdal may cause Neuroleptic Malignant Syndrome (NMS), a condition marked by muscle stiffness or rigidity, fast heartbeat or irregular pulse, increased sweating, high fever, and high or low blood pressure. Unchecked, this condition can prove fatal.

Patients at high risk for suicide attempts will be prescribed the lowest dose possible to reduce the risk of intentional overdose.

The safety and effectiveness of Risperdal in children have not been established.

Common side effects[14]: Abdominal pain, abnormal walk, agitation, aggression, anxiety, chest pain, constipation, coughing, decreased activity, diarrhea, dizziness, dry skin, fever, headache, inability to sleep, increased dreaming, increased duration of sleep, indigestion, involuntary movements, joint pain, lack of coordination, nasal inflammation, nausea, overactivity, rapid heartbeat, rash, reduced salivation, respiratory infection, sleepiness, sore throat, tremor, underactive reflexes, urination problems, vomiting, weight gain.

■

Our sole intent in seeking medical help all along had been to set Jeff on a "normal" path. Since he was so young, there wasn't much empirical evidence to go on. It was only in retrospect that we viewed the full course of his treatment as a grand medical ex-

---

13 This is an abridged description of Risperdal taken from http://www.pdrhealth.com, the official online patient resource based on the PDR (Copyright ©2003 Thomson Healthcare).

14 For more complete information, see www.pdrhealth.com, another reliable medical reference source, or ask your physician.

periment. The number of different medications Jeff was on had reached alarming proportions. I had always been under the impression that decisions were to be made jointly between doctor and parent; the doctor was the expert, but the family had the hands-on experience. Together, I hoped we would be able to determine which medications would be used and for what reasons—I needed to trust the doctor. But instead, the rate at which drugs were being prescribed and changed had become a marathon of confusion and fear for me. Decisions were so crucial, but I didn't feel qualified in many ways to make them.

The drugs prescribed for Jeffrey did have successful track records; unfortunately, few of them were considered appropriate for a child his age, and they all had potential for such alarming side effects. There were several times when doctors ignored my suggestions and concerns completely, and made me feel like an idiot by expounding their qualifications and experience versus mine. I actually had very little say when it came down to a disagreement about treatment—the doctor was always right.

Chapter 6

B Y FEBRUARY 1999, WHEN Jeffrey was five, I was desperate. I made the decision to move to Washington State to be near my brother and his family. At the time, it seemed like a good idea to relocate so that my brother's family could be more involved in Jeffrey's life, and so that I could help my sister-in-law, who was ill. I could also give my parents their lives back.

There were no solutions for Jeffrey there, either. Under our insurance plan, there was not a psychiatrist within driving distance who would take Jeffrey on—his case was too complex. Finally, a pediatrician referred us to a child psychiatrist and we were accepted into Catholic Community Services, a mental health service for low-income families with extreme needs. Between the move and the lapse in services, Jeffrey's behavior steadily declined. The move was not good in terms of his schooling, either. At Jeffrey's new kindergarten, they provided a one-on-one aide, but it was mostly to protect the other children. His first field trip was his last, and Jeff was banned from riding the school bus after he threatened to kill another child by cutting off his head. He also told me that the robots were back in his stomach.

As with all relationships with Jeffrey, it didn't take long for my brother's family to realize the impossibility of living a normal life with him around. Jeffrey is like a dripping faucet—at first, it's a little annoying; but the longer it drips, the fuller the sink, and the louder the drips, the bigger the splash! My brother feared for his own son's safety. I was disappointed, but I certainly didn't blame them. At the end of six months, we moved back to California.

The non-public SED school Jeffrey had attended before we moved to Washington now had no openings. The school district placed Jeff in a regular public school in an SED classroom until another IEP could be held.

Tegretol[1] (brand name)

Generic name: Carbamazepine

Other brand names: Carbatrol, Epitol

Indications: Tegretol is used in the treatment of seizure disorders, including certain types of epilepsy. It is also prescribed for trigeminal neuralgia (severe pain in the jaws) and pain in the tongue and throat. Some doctors also prescribe Tegretol to treat alcohol withdrawal, cocaine addiction, and emotional disorders such as depression and abnormally aggressive behavior. The drug may be used to treat migraine headache and "restless legs."

Warnings: There are potentially dangerous side effects associated with the use of Tegretol. Symptoms such as fever, sore throat, rash, ulcers in the mouth, easy bruising, or reddish or purplish spots on the skin could be signs of a blood disorder brought on by the drug. You should notify your doctor.

Common side effects[2]: abnormal heartbeat and rhythm, abnormal involuntary movements, aching joints and muscles, agitation, anemia, blood clots, blurred vision, chills, congestive heart failure, depression, dizziness, drowsiness, nausea, vomiting, double vision, dry mouth and throat, fainting and collapse, fatigue, fever, fluid retention, hallucinations, headache, hepatitis, hives, inflamed eyes, itching, kidney failure, leg cramps, liver disorders, loss of appetite, low blood pressure, pancreatitis (inflammation of the pancreas), pneumonia, reddened skin, ringing in the ears, sensitivity to light, sensitivity to sound, skin inflammation and scaling, peeling, rashes, or pigmentation changes, speech difficulties, stomach problems, sweating, talkativeness, tingling sensation, worsening of high blood pressure, yellow eyes and skin

---

1 This is an abridged description of Tegretol taken from the Physician's Desk Reference (PDR) as it appears at http://www.pdrhealth.com, the official online patient resource based on the PDR (Copyright ©2003 Thomson Healthcare).

2 For more complete information, see www.pdrhealth.com, another reliable medical reference source, or ask your physician.

The county office of education referred us to a program called "Wrap Around," which was part of immediate mental health services. They were to provide counselors, behavior specialists, and psychiatrists for Jeff as often as needed to keep him from harming himself and others. During that first month of school, his behavior deteriorated even more rapidly despite the help he was receiving, so the county psychiatrist added yet another medication—Tegretol. A week later, it was recommended that Jeffrey be admitted to a local psychiatric hospital for fourteen days. Those two weeks seemed like an eternity. We were only allowed to visit for an hour each evening—those were the program's rules. Meanwhile, medications were swapped and changed and tried for the first time in an attempt to find something that would help.

At the hospital, Jeffrey was described as: "extremely difficult to redirect, very mean with other children, kicking blocks down, hitting, interrupting, and being very critical." His nickname there was Bam-Bam—he was strong, blond, and he hit everything. Jeff had been very slim until the age of five; then, he'd ballooned up to 86 pounds due to the medications he was taking. He could not eat enough food, and seemed to be transfixed by eating. A doctor at the hospital described his eating as almost ritualistic—as if the act put him into a trance. He would shut his eyes and shovel enormous quantities of food into his mouth at one sitting.

Gradually, he was learning to hone his manipulation techniques. He always wanted to be first in line, and to answer questions first. "In general," the staff reported, "he is somewhat bossy."

Many ADHD and behaviorally challenged children are extremely intelligent. Jeff is no exception. His teachers have consistently commented about his abilities and his impressive vocabulary—his testing also reflects this. To talk to him, anyone would assume that he was much older than his biological years. Jeff thought so far ahead of every situation, his counselors at a residential program declared him to be a "master manipulator," and said that he was, "able to orchestrate charisma." Jeffrey has always been adorable; he's a handsome kid, and he knows how to charm. He could wing his way through most any situation, as long as he didn't lose control. Jeffrey could turn words inside out and upside down until the truth became obscured.

Adderall and Mellaril were reintroduced, as the Risperdal was not effective. I vehemently objected, as Mellaril had always increased his hostility in the past, and Adderall had shown no appreciable benefits. They elected to do it anyway, while gradually decreasing the Risperdal.

At the end of the two weeks, I was informed by the hospital staff that Jeffrey would be discharged. The doctor apologized, explaining that his insurance only covered a certain number of days. There was little regard for Jeff's state of health. Insurance in general had always added to our problems. Jeff had been covered by military insurance for most of his years, but it was secondary to any other coverage he might have. For many years, because of my low-income status, I had been able to get him coverage through a state program, though we did not qualify for welfare because I owned a car.

Jeff's discharge summary read: "Two days after initiating the Mellaril, the patient became quite a bit more whiny, with no frustration tolerance at all. He was not aggressive to other children but he simply would fall down on the floor, screaming and crying if he did not get what he wanted. It was very difficult to calm him. His mother was convinced that this was from the Mellaril and I tend to agree. As we were approaching discharge, and the patient prior to the Mellaril had been doing relatively well, we elected to stop the Mellaril at the time of discharge. At discharge, the mother, who had requested that the patient be taken off all medications at the beginning of hospitalization, was still eager to do this as he had been on medications for two years. This was sanctioned by myself and the mother was told how to gradually decrease the Tegratol and the Risperdal."

We removed Jeffrey from the hospital with great trepidation. We all knew it was too soon to release him but we had no other choice. My father came along to help physically control Jeff on the drive home. It was heartbreaking—Jeff thrashed and fought the whole way.

The child psychiatrist at the hospital had recommended that Jeffrey be placed in a highly supervised school classroom with a small teacher/child ratio and the capacity to work closely with outpatient clinicians and psychiatrists. The IEP process had started in August 1999 and by the time Jeffrey was released from the hospital in September, the IEP had been completed. Their recommendation was to start Jeff in a new non-public, day treatment school in a nearby community. The therapeutic clinician and psychiatrist from the Wrap Around service would continue to support the family.

The day after his discharge, I took Jeffrey to meet with a Wrap Around service psychiatrist who had seen Jeffrey once before. I was adamant, arguing that Jeffrey should be taken off all medications. I refused to fill any prescriptions. After thirty minutes of debate, his insistent optimism persuaded me to at least give his treatment recommendations a chance. He stressed that he had seen children like Jeffrey before, and he had successfully treated them with medication. He convinced me that I should trust his experience and expertise.

With the assurance that Jeff just had to get used to the medicines again, the doctor gave me a note I have saved to this day: "There will be a light at the end of this tunnel!" He also wrote down exactly what medications Jeff needed and when to give them to him: They were:

Risperdal 3 mg, 1 am, 1 pm

Seroquel 100 mg, 1 3x a day

Neurontin 300 mg, 1 4 x a day

Tegretol 200 mg, 1 3x a day

Klonopin was to be given when Jeff was out of control: 1 mg, 1 tablet every 8 hours. The doctor told me, "I am experienced, I have seen this before, we can beat it! It will be tough, and it may get worse before it gets better." He repeated, "but there is a light at the end of the tunnel!"

Seroquel[3] (brand name)

Generic name: Quetiapine fumarate

Indications: Seroquel is the first in a new class of antipsychotic medications used to combat the symptoms of schizophrenia. Researchers believe that it works by diminishing the action of dopamine and serotonin, two of the brain's chief chemical messengers.

Warnings: Seroquel may cause tardive dyskinesia--a condition characterized by uncontrollable muscle spasms and twitches in the face and body. This problem can be permanent, and appears to be most common among older adults, especially women.

Side effects of muscle stiffness, confusion, irregular or rapid heartbeat, excessive sweating, and high fever are signs of a serious--and potentially fatal--reaction to the drug. Contact your doctor immediately.

Common side effects[4]: Abdominal pain, constipation, diminished movement, dizziness, drowsiness, dry mouth, excessive muscle tone, headache, indigestion, low blood pressure, nasal inflammation, neck rigidity, rapid heartbeat, rash, tremor, uncontrollable movements, weakness

---

3 This is an abridged description of Seroquel taken from the Physician's Desk Reference (PDR) as it appears at http://www.pdrhealth.com, the official online patient resource based on the PDR (©2003 Thomson Healthcare).

4 For more complete information, see www.pdrhealth.com, another reliable medical reference source, or ask your physician.

Neurontin[5] (brand name)

Generic name: Gabapentin

Indications: Neurontin may be prescribed with other medications to treat partial seizures. It can be used whether or not the seizures eventually become general and result in loss of consciousness. It can also be used to relieve the burning nerve pain that sometimes persists after an attack of shingles (herpes zoster).

Warnings: In children, Neurontin occasionally triggers behavioral problems such as unstable emotions, hostility, aggression, hyperactivity, and lack of concentration. However, such problems (if they occur) are usually mild.

Common side effects[6]: When taken for epilepsy, more common side effects include: blurred, dimmed, or double vision, bronchitis (in children), dizziness, drowsiness, fatigue, fever (in children), involuntary eye movement, itchy, runny nose, lack of muscular coordination, nausea, tremor, viral infection (in children), vomiting, weight increase (in children)

When taken for nerve pain, more common side effects include: accidental injury, constipation, diarrhea, dizziness, drowsiness, dry mouth, headache, infection, lack of muscular coordination, nausea, swelling in arms and legs, vomiting, weakness

A wide variety of uncommon and rare side effects have also been reported. If you develop any new or unusual symptoms while taking Neurontin, be sure to let your doctor know.

■

That next week was nothing short of hellish, but the doctor's professional optimism was like waving a life preserver over the head of a drowning victim. He gave me hope. Despite the exhausting week, I told my mom that I had finally found a doctor who promised he could help Jeffrey. That hope was short lived.

At the day treatment facility, Jeffrey rode on a supervised bus that picked him up and returned him home each day. The program there included group and individual therapy and psychiatric monitoring—it was a much more intensive therapeutic regi-

---

5 This is an abridged description of Neurontin taken from the Physician's Desk Reference (PDR) as it appears at http://www.pdrhealth.com, the official online patient resource based on the PDR (©2003 Thomson Healthcare).

6 For more complete information, see www.pdrhealth.com, another reliable medical reference source, or ask your physician.

men than he had ever had. The "light at the end of the tunnel" doctor was supportive and encouraging. No doctor had ever displayed such optimism about Jeffrey's future. We held our collective breath waiting for any positive results. There didn't appear to be any changes for the better. By this time, this doctor had started Jeffrey on five different medications and the side effects were jaw dropping.

Klonopin[7] (brand name)

Generic name: Clonazepam

Indications: Klonopin is used alone or with other medications to treat convulsive disorders such as epilepsy. It is also prescribed for panic disorder--unexpected attacks of overwhelming panic accompanied by fear of recurrence. Klonopin belongs to a class of drugs known as benzodiazepines.

Warnings: If you have several types of seizures, this drug may increase the possibility of grand mal seizures (epilepsy).

Klonopin can be habit-forming and can lose its effectiveness as you build up a tolerance to it.

For panic disorder, safety and effectiveness have not been established in children under age 18.

Common side effects[8]: Klonopin can cause aggressive behavior, agitation, anxiety, excitability, hostility, irritability, nervousness, nightmares, sleep disturbances, and vivid dreams. In panic disorder side effects may include: Allergic reaction, constipation, coordination problems, depression, dizziness, fatigue, inflamed sinuses or nasal passages, flu, memory problems, menstrual problems, nervousness, reduced thinking ability, respiratory infection, sleepiness, speech problems

∎

One morning, a week after the meds were started, I found Jeffrey to be very lethargic and uncoordinated. He could barely walk—he was tripping over his own feet and falling down—but

---

7 This is an abridged description of Klonopin taken from the Physician's Desk Reference (PDR) as it appears at http://www.pdrhealth.com, the official online patient resource based on the PDR (©2003 Thomson Healthcare).

8 For more complete information, see www.pdrhealth.com, another reliable medical reference source, or ask your physician.

I couldn't help him because he was so volatile and combative. Finally, I got him in the car and drove to my parents' home. Jeffrey stumbled into the house, waving his arms around and yelling. He climbed up onto my mother's lap, and to our utter surprise, he calmed down almost immediately. She gently held him while I called the doctor, her eyes filling with tears as he tried to talk— jumbled words that made no sense spilled out. Then we noticed a large wet spot growing on her shoulder—Jeffrey was drooling.

When I described Jeffrey's condition to the doctor, he insisted we take him directly to a local psychiatric hospital. He also instructed us to give him another dose of Clonazepam to subdue him until we could get him to the hospital. Thank heavens for maternal instinct: I chose not to give him any more. I learned later that it could have been lethal. In the end, the "light at the end of the tunnel" ended up being far too close to the white light that people describe seeing during a near-death experience. We had maintained hope right up until the time Jeffrey was admitted for a second time to the psychiatric hospital. He had been so mismedicated and overmedicated that he could barely function, yet he remained as violent and dangerous as he'd ever been. We could not see any light at the end of the tunnel that loomed ahead—instead it appeared dark, long, and very frightening.

Jeffrey was at the psychatric hospital for 10 days this time, and was immediately put through a protocol of detoxification. He was then sent home without any medication, sanctioning my belief that none of these drugs were working anyway. His discharge papers stated: "Jeffrey's behavior had escalated, in spite of, or because of, the additional medications. He was weaned off all medication over the first part of his admission and his behavior became less tense, less aggressive and he became more cooperative. He continues to be quite hyperactive. The doctors elected to do a trial of stimulant medication and put him on Adderall for two days.

Each day he was irritable and more aggressive, cried frequently, and had no frustration tolerance. We elected to stop Adderall, and he settled down a bit. It is our impression that the patient at this point in time does best on no medication. He requires a highly structured environment, both at school and at home, with a high level of supervision. At discharge the patient was manageable but required supervision. He was not suicidal and was not hearing any voices and was looking forward to going home and back to his new school."

Jeff was again returned to the day treatment facility, where they worked closely with him and tried to keep his aggression under control. Within weeks, it was clear that nothing was going to keep him from posing a danger to himself or to others. His behavior decreased to the point where, in December 1999, he started kicking staff, being aggressive toward peers, overreacting, badgering, and having space issues and problems in the school van. He violently attacked a cat at school, kicking it repeatedly. The school recommended hospitalization for re-evaluation, and Jeffrey was readmitted to the psych hospital from December 6th to December 11th, 1999. Jeffrey remained free of medication during this hospital visit, but his mental and behavioral state continued to be very unstable.

As a condition of his discharge, the hospital placed Jeff in a 90-day residential evaluation program. This local facility was large, with quite a few children housed together in groups. After 30 days he was moved to a unit with fewer children, but he continued to demonstrate extreme aggression. Jeffrey remained there until February 17, 2001. We were only allowed to visit him occasionally and take him to doctor appointments. At the end of this period, it was determined that he needed residential placement to allow round-the-clock therapeutic care. He was transferred to a Boys' Ranch 50 miles from our home. His services were upgraded to those of a therapeutic residential program; this time, Jeffrey would actually

Oppositional Defiance Disorder[9] (ODD)

Children and teens with this disorder are hostile toward their parents or other authority figures. They often argue about rules and may break them. Other characteristics of people with ODD include losing their temper, annoying others on purpose, blaming others for their mistakes or misbehavior, being overly sensitive, and possibly angry, resentful, or vengeful. Defiance is fairly common in all children, especially in teenagers. Before a diagnosis of ODD can be made, it needs to persist over six months. It can cause significant problems within the family.

- Almost half of children and teens with Attention Deficit Hyperactivity Disorder (ADHD) also have Oppositional Defiance Disorder.

- Oppositional defiance will worsen to Conduct Disorder in some children and teens. Children with Conduct Disorder may have a pattern of lying, stealing, and cheating, may skip school or run away from home, and may harm animals, property, and other people.

live there. He was six years old and one of the youngest children at the Ranch.

Our home was certainly more peaceful, but the emptiness was overpowering. We all felt numb. Relative to the constant barrage of noise that always accompanied Jeff, the house was miserably silent. We had to remind ourselves over and over that it was a crucial matter of safety, of saving Jeff's life. Still, we were frightened for him, and nervous about his adjustment to the Ranch. We prayed they were keeping a 24-hour vigil over him. I wandered the house alone at night, wondering if he was okay, if he missed me, if he was scared. Regardless of his problems, I wanted my son with me.

9 WebMd.com, © 1995-2004, Healthwise, Incorporated, P.O. Box 1989, Boise, ID 83701.

Chapter 7

THE STAY AT THE Boys' Ranch didn't last long. Even in this highly supervised and therapeutic residential care program, Jeffrey's behavior was deteriorating. Nightly phone calls and visits home over the weekends were privileges that he had to earn through good behavior. I drove the 50 miles to the Ranch twice a week, once for individual therapy and once for family therapy. Jeff was occasionally able to attend the family therapy. Other than that, we only saw him on the weekends when his behavior merited the reward. The longer he was there, the less we got to see him. If he couldn't come home for the weekend, we would go see him and take him to lunch or to a movie. Even telephone contact became less frequent as time went on. My parents and I took turns calling, but as his behavior spiraled downward, so did his opportunities to talk to us.

I was able to get more sleep, hold down a job, and I could actually take a shower or bath at my leisure, but I missed my little boy so much. I felt such a deep sense of hurt for him, knowing his childhood had already been full of so many nightmarish experiences. Now he was at a place where he never got the loving reassurance of a nite-nite hug, or "smoochies" as we called them; there was no one there to tell him, "I love you."

Jeff's behavior deteriorated to the point that he was moved to a room by himself, and was required to wear a swimming suit to take his daily shower because he had to be accompanied by an adult attendant at all times. Because of his escalating aggression, the doctor felt it appropriate to start him on pharmaceuticals again, and the roller coaster began its ascent. He had been off medication for three months when Ritalin was reintroduced, specifically for hyperactivity. I agreed because I could see he wasn't getting any better. Trying medication that had already failed to produce results seemed foolhardy, but the doctors seemed to think that the change in environment, or a change in combined pharmaceuticals might yield different or more promising results. No pharmaceutical we'd tried, alone or in combination, had helped yet—there was no magic bullet. The most I dared to hope for was a halt to Jeff's terrifying decline.

Six weeks later, Jeffrey exhibited symptoms of severe depression. The psychiatrist called and reported to me that he would be prescribing the antidepressant Clonazepam (Klonopin). Again, I agreed, but I reminded him that Jeffrey hadn't responded well to Clonazepam in the past. Two weeks later, the doctor called again to tell me he felt Jeff was suicidal. Now he wanted to change the antidepressant to Zoloft. In October, Neurontin was added, because Jeff had not responded as expected to any of the medications.

That was the worst Christmas of our lives. Jeff lost his phone privileges—we couldn't talk to him at all. He lost all visitation privileges, too. He was not able to leave the facility for six weeks leading up to Christmas 2000. A holiday party was held for families, and my parents and I were thrilled to be able to see him, but on Christmas Day, Jeff was not allowed to come home. I was benevolently allowed a two-hour visit in the therapy room with him instead. Hoping to make it as special as I possibly could, I went overboard. I bought him everything I knew he wanted: decks and decks of Pokemon cards, a Razor scooter, and Legos, amongst a multitude of other things. Jeff opened each and every gift and complained—nothing was the right color, it was a duplicate, it was just plain wrong. He was completely dissatisfied. At first, I was heartbroken—until I got angry. I really let loose that day. It was the year Jeffrey learned who Santa really was. He was so ungrateful and abusive, shouting, "You should have done better! You never do anything for me!" I drove home in tears—my special Christmas had been disastrous.

Zoloft[1] (brand name)

Generic name: Sertraline

Indications: Zoloft is a member of the family of drugs called "selective serotonin re-uptake inhibitors (SSRI)." It is prescribed for major depressive disorder—a persistently low mood that interferes with everyday living. Zoloft is also used for the treatment of obsessive-compulsive disorder, panic disorder, premenstrual dysphoric disorder (PMDD), and posttraumatic stress disorder.

Warnings: If you have a kidney or liver disorder, or are subject to seizures, take Zoloft cautiously and under close medical supervision.

In a few people, Zoloft may trigger the grandiose, inappropriate, out-of-control behavior called mania or the similar, but less dramatic, "hyper" state called hypomania.

Safety and effectiveness have not been established for children under 6.

Common side effects[2]: Abdominal pain, agitation, anxiety, constipation, diarrhea or loose stools, dizziness, dry mouth, fatigue, gas, headache, decreased appetite, increased sweating, indigestion, insomnia, nausea, nervousness, pain, rash, sleepiness, sore throat, tingling or pins and needles, tremor, vision problems, vomiting

Zoloft may also cause mental or emotional symptoms such as: Abnormal dreams or thoughts, aggressiveness, exaggerated feeling of well-being, depersonalization ("unreal" feeling), hallucinations, impaired concentration, memory loss, paranoia, rapid mood shifts, suicidal thoughts, tooth-grinding, worsened depression

---

1 This is an abridged description of Zoloft taken from the Physician's Desk Reference (PDR) as it appears at www.pdrhealth.com, the official online patient resource based on the PDR (©2003 Thomson Healthcare).

2 For more complete information, see www.pdrhealth.com, another reliable medical reference source, or ask your physician.

Like a lead anchor, everything was sinking. I could tell he was now doing things purposely to fail. The school psychologist reported that, "overall, Jeffrey's poor behavior negatively impacted his academic progress because Jeffrey was always doing something to remove himself from the class. His behaviors ranged from shouting in class to demonstrating extreme physical aggression, kicking adults in the shins, hitting in the groin, and scratching at someone's face with his nails, according to his teacher. His aggression was usually targeting adults in the environment because he wasn't given the opportunity to harm his peers, requiring one-on-one attention from an adult at all times." He had been in their care for seven months, and his behavior was worse than ever.

Since none of his peers ever wanted to be around him for long, and because he knew he'd been asked to leave so many schools, he had always wanted to fit in and be part of the group. But his way of fitting in never worked, because he also needed to be the boss. He insisted on hitting the first and the last ball, he made up the rules, picked the teams, and chose the game. He was by himself almost constantly as a result—alone and angry.

Jeffrey continued to speak often about killing himself and others. He was placed on suicide watch, with an attendant posted outside his bedroom door each night. Reportedly, he tied a shirt around his neck one night; on another occasion, he had wrapped his bathrobe tie around his throat. This was such a low point in his life: he was hated by his peers, adults shunned him, he had no father, he was separated from us, and he was all alone. I could relate to a degree—I'd mentally beaten myself up often, wondering how I had failed him so miserably. I don't believe Jeffrey ever really wanted to end his life—I think he was just so lonely and sad, he wanted attention, however it came.

The situation became so charged at the Ranch that that there was talk of the other boys "getting Jeffrey," whatever that meant. We knew his days were numbered. We received the phone call we were dreading on February 8th, 2001. They gave us seven days to find another placement for him, declaring him more than they could handle. They were at a loss—he had to have one-on-one attention, even when showering and sleeping.

At this type of facility, the severity of a child's behavioral problems was classified by "levels." This made sense to us—we absolutely agreed that every child there needed adequate supervision. Levels had increasing requirements for supervision and therapy. The higher the level, the more staff needed to meet the more intense therapy and supervision guidelines. This facility was classified as a Level 12, which meant that they had one adult supervisor for every three to four students. It was decided that Jeff required a Level 14 facility, which had one adult for every one to two students. Jeff's violence was causing the staff to fear for their own safety, and for the well being of the other boys there. After days of extensive research on both my part and county staff, we learned there were no higher-level residential care facilities or programs in the entire state of California that would accept a child as young as Jeffrey. It was decided that Jeffrey would be placed on Independent Study until a Level 14 placement could be secured.

A county meeting was held on Valentine's Day. The family, probation, County Board of Education members, county mental health workers, CALWORKS, and the heads of all the county departments that could contribute to the situation were present. Referred to as a "case conference," the outcome consisted of recommendations that might allow Jeffrey to avoid a Level 14 designation and remain living at home, but with a more comprehensive approach to therapy. Specifically, we would explore the following points:

1 Jeffrey would return home with one-on-one behavioral help
2 He would continue mental health services

3 The family team, who were all case workers, would set up additional support services

4 Jeff would possibly take part in the Riding High equestrian therapy program

5 He would have an individualized exercise program

6 Jeff and I would seek an alternative living situation (preferably in the country)

7 We would continue the exploration of medication

8 I would stop working and receive funding in order to be available full-time for Jeffrey's care, a notion referred to as "performance instead of dollars"

We were to reconvene at the upcoming IEP on the 16th of February. The group seemed to be excited that I still wanted to be involved in Jeffrey's recovery, and that I was not ready to "give him up to the system." I was excited that there seemed to be so many avenues of help available, and that everyone was on board and even considering alternative treatments. A home hospital teacher would visit with him for one hour a day, and I would quit my job as a high school teacher's aide to be home full-time with him. We also agreed that I would find living arrangements that were not part of an apartment complex because on previous occasions, the police had been called to investigate all the noise coming from our apartment. After that, we had filed a form at the local police department describing the situation so that we could avoid any future misunderstandings. The preference was for Jeff and I to live in the country, where he could run free and avoid distractions, but funding wasn't available and living so far from immediate help scared me. I found a home to rent, the IEP team offered to pay me what I had been earning, and they would provide in-home support.

I brought Jeffrey home on February 16, 2001. We were still in the apartment the first time the home hospital teacher came to work with him. She wrote in her report that day: "Jeffrey would not acknowledge me when I walked into the room. He would not answer any questions. He stated that he did not need to go to school and wouldn't go to school. Jeffrey acted defiant and stated that he wanted to kill himself with the pencils. He threw the pencils at the wall." She refused to come back.

Zyprexa[3] (brand name)

Generic name: Olanzapine

Indications: Zyprexa helps manage symptoms of schizophrenia, the manic phase of manic-depression, and other psychotic disorders.

Warnings: At the start of Zyprexa therapy, the drug can cause extreme low blood pressure, increased heart rate, dizziness, and, in rare cases, a tendency to faint when first standing up. These problems are more likely if you are dehydrated, have heart disease, or take blood pressure medicine.

Zyprexa sometimes causes drowsiness and can impair your judgment, thinking, and motor skills.

Medicines such as Zyprexa can interfere with regulation of the body's temperature. Do not get overheated or become dehydrated while taking Zyprexa.

Drugs such as Zyprexa sometimes cause a condition called Neuroleptic Malignant Syndrome. Symptoms include high fever, muscle rigidity, irregular pulse or blood pressure, rapid heartbeat, excessive perspiration, and changes in heart rhythm.

There is also a risk of developing tardive dyskinesia, a condition marked by slow, rhythmical, involuntary movements.

Zyprexa contains phenylalanine, so children with phenylketonuria should not take this drug.

Common side effects[4]: Abdominal pain, abnormal gait, agitation, anxiety, back pain, blood in urine, blurred vision, chest pain, constipation, cough, dehydration, dizziness, drowsiness, dry mouth, extreme low blood pressure, eye problems, fever, headache, high blood pressure, hostility, increased appetite, indigestion, inflammation of the nasal passages and throat, insomnia, joint pain, movement disorders, muscle rigidity, nausea, nervousness, rapid heartbeat, tension, tremor, weight gain

---

3 This is an abridged description of Zyprexa taken from the Physician's Desk Reference (PDR) as it appears at www.pdrhealth.com, the official online patient resource based on the PDR (Copyright ©2003 Thomson Healthcare).

4 For more complete information, see www.pdrhealth.com, another reliable medical reference source, or ask your physician.

At the IEP, I had been informed that Jeffrey would be seeing the county psychiatrist. I wasn't too happy about it—I had already had several run-ins with him and we had disagreed about medications. At our first appointment, he immediately suggested Imipramine, which had previously failed Jeffrey while under this same doctor's care at the county SED school less than two years ago. I objected and stood my ground—No Imipramine. He reluctantly agreed to try a new drug—Zyprexa. I insisted that if after four weeks there was no positive result, I wanted Jeffrey removed from the medication. We saw the doctor two weeks later, when he gave us a handful of other prescriptions to add to the Zyprexa, all of which Jeffrey had been on at one time or another. I firmly reminded him that they had already proven to be ineffective and I would not allow him to be put on those drugs again. I was mystified by the fact that doctor after doctor was recommending the same prescriptions that had failed Jeffrey in the past, as if they were a brand new solution.

When I left his office, I immediately contacted the mental health case worker and told her that I would not subject my son to any additional medications, and that I wanted him to be weaned off the Zyprexa. I felt that the doctor was prescribing more drugs than were necessary, and that the Zyprexa was not working. She said she would talk to the doctor, but suggested that I contact him as well. I tried calling him several times—he did not return my calls. I went to a pre-planned appointment with him; I had taken Jeffrey out of school early to get there on time. When we arrived, the doctor said he would just be a minute. After ten minutes, the secretary assured me that the doctor wouldn't be long; after 20 minutes, and with Jeffrey's short attention span well spent, I had his secretary write a note stating that I would be removing Jeffrey from all of his medication and if he had any concerns, to contact me immediately. We left and never heard from him again.

For a very short while, Jeffrey was off all medications and was relatively happy to be living at home. He started at the non-public school for emotionally and behaviorally challenged children in March 2001. He was not allowed to ride the bus for fear he would harm another child. Therefore, I transported him to and from school every day, a 75-mile round trip.

County and social services agents were in and out of our home every day. I had daily, weekly, and monthly meetings, parenting classes, and behavioral modification courses; Jeffrey had after-school activities, therapy, behavioral counseling, and so on. Some avenues of help had fallen away. Even with the commitment of assistance from the latest IEP, it was obvious that Jeffrey needed more care and intervention than we were collectively able to provide. In May 2001, another IEP was called. We discussed the failures of our previous plan, and were given 30 days to come up with another strategy, or his care level would be increased to Level 14 care. This meant I would be forced to place him in an out-of-state facility with this level of available care.

At this point, we had exhausted so many options. Jeff's medical charts looked like a crazy experiment. At seven years old, he had been asked to leave every school he had attended, he had been treated by sixteen different doctors, and he had been on at least sixteen psychotropic drugs (alone or in combination). He had been admitted on three separate occasions to a psychiatric hospital. When one drug didn't seem to help, or if it made things worse, another drug would be introduced to help counteract the side effects of the first drug. When that didn't help, yet another drug would be added to the mix, or the dosages would be changed.

When do you say enough is enough? When do you tell all the "professionals" that you think they are actually harming your child, and that you fear for his life? When do you let go of that little piece of hope that you will find that one therapy or doctor or medicine that will finally make a difference? It was like riding a roller coaster: you climb up and up hoping against hope, you teeter on the brink, full of expectation and a little fear, and then suddenly you are over the edge, crashing back to where you'd started. Then, you catch a glimpse of yet another mountain of hope to climb. When do you jump off the roller coaster? When do you abandon hope for your child?

Chapter 8

WHEN I AGREED TO quit my job in order to care for Jeffrey full time, I had been working for less than a year as an instructional aide for special needs teens at a local high school. I love teenagers, and they have always responded very well to me. Not long before I left the position, my students presented a debate in speech class on marijuana and its use as a medication. Up until then, I'd been completely in the dark about the subject. I had never used marijuana; I didn't know anyone who did (or so I thought!); and my family and I were conservative Christians who had voted against Proposition 215, which passed in 1996, legalizing marijuana for medicinal use in the state of California. We had never bothered to learn about marijuana, and frankly, at first, we were not open to even exploring it as a possible treatment for Jeffrey. Any exposure we'd had to marijuana was what we'd gotten from the mainstream media. Our general view was that "pot," "dope," "grass"—whatever you wanted to call it—was part of a counterculture movement that didn't have much value.

Religion didn't have anything to do with our views about marijuana. It was the legality of the issue that was foremost in our minds. Marijuana was categorized as an illicit substance. Through my students' reports, however, I was amazed to learn that marijuana had been used to treat mental disorders, and many other ailments, dating back to ancient times! My first impulse was to dismiss this notion, but I was also intrigued. A little voice in the back of my head urged me to set aside my prejudices until I had more information. It certainly wouldn't hurt to educate myself by doing a little research.

When we had exhausted so many other options and were facing the prospect of Jeffrey being sent to an out-of-state program, I stepped up my research. I wanted to find out if marijuana had any potential as a medicine for Jeffrey. I asked to see the material my young debaters had come up with, I spoke with friends who were somewhat knowledgeable about the subject, and I began doing extensive Internet investigation. My questions were endless, yet I hardly knew where to begin. What was the history of this plant? What were the side effects of using it as medicine? How was it administered? I wanted to know more about the details of Proposition 215 and all of the legal issues involved.

I understood that as a Californian, Jeffrey had a legal right to use medical marijuana if recommended by his physician under Prop. 215. But what physicians would be open to considering such a recommendation? How would they determine if Jeffrey was a suitable candidate? And if he was, where would the marijuana be obtained? Would I have to grow it myself? Certainly he wouldn't be smoking the stuff, would he?

I researched every book I could find on the subject—they ran the gamut from rebellious and cartoonish to serious and backed by empirical evidence. I scoured the Internet: some sites seemed on the up and up and some appeared to be a little shady. I stuck with the sites that were presented by seemingly caring, science-driven persons—botanists, scientists, and doctors. Even after all this research, I couldn't make an immediate decision to act until I had spoken with our family physician and several doctors, the county support team (who snickered a bit), the county educational team, several teachers, countless Internet contacts, my parents, and a close family friend who had used marijuana. I made a conscious effort to be very open about telling people that I was considering medical marijuana for Jeffrey. In general, I wanted to learn more about the implications for him, and I certainly didn't want to appear to be hiding anything. I had to keep reminding myself that it was legal.

To my surprise, the general consensus across the board was a big "thumbs up" on going forward with this "medical exploration." Anyone who knew me could rest assured that I would only do what was best for Jeffrey. Nothing had worked in the past; even the doctors knew that. With the 30-day deadline looming, it seemed to me that we should explore any alternatives we had left. Not a single person warned me against using marijuana, or appeared alarmed by the suggestion.

My parents, in fact, were the only holdouts—they thought I was crazy. Mom and Dad believed that marijuana use was unlawful and foolhardy—they weren't aware yet of what marijuana's applications as a medicine were. They could not shake their preconceived notions of marijuana as something for "stoners." I shared all of my information with them. At least they listened. My mother held her position, though. At an IEP meeting where I formally announced my decision to put Jeffrey on a trial of medical marijuana as recommended by a doctor, my mother was so upset she left the room without a word. She feared repercussions, and was convinced that we should keep our plans to ourselves, at least until after we knew whether it would work or not. I disagreed: I felt that keeping secrets would be problematic in the long run. I wasn't doing anything wrong.

As I continued to share my research with my mother, her skepticism began to turn into interest and very cautious hope. Soon, even she had to admit that medical marijuana was far less harmful than any of the medications that had already been prescribed for Jeffrey. In fact, I discovered that all of the medications Jeffrey had taken in the past had far greater potential risks than the medical marijuana. According to the Physician's Desk Reference (PDR) these medications:

- are not recommended for children his age
- their safety and effectiveness in children has not been established
- they could cause severe liver damage
- they could stunt a child's growth
- they could cause permanent muscle problems
- they are highly addictive
- they are lethal in an overdose

None of Jeff's drugs had been proven safe nor effective for children; that was the fact. Here was a drug with few, if any, side effects, which he had not been treated with—yet. There were multitudes of anecdotal examples of how it had helped people with psychotic, assaultive aggressive behaviors and Obsessive Compulsive Disorder (OCD). When the wide array of drugs we'd already tried were reviewed solely on the basis of side effects and toxicity, the contraindications were appalling, especially as compared to marijuana.

I was very interested to see marijuana (listed as "cannabis") in the PDR as well: "No health hazards or side effects are known in conjunction with the proper administration of designated therapeutic dosages of medical marijuana. The intake of toxic dosages, as is common with the smoking of cannabis, leads almost at once to euphoric states (pronounced gaiety, laughing fits)."

Apparently, an overdose of medical marijuana could cause a bad case of the giggles, but nowhere did it say it had the potential to damage your liver, stunt your growth, make you drool, or kill you. I had tried to keep an open mind about sixteen other drugs, so why not this one? I was open to any legal and ethical solution. In the end, the choice was crystal clear.

Determined now to go ahead with my decision, I had to find a reliable, responsible, understanding, and absolutely legal source of help. I sat down in front of the computer and typed the words "compassion and marijuana" into the Internet search engine. The results included a link to a site called WAMM (Wo/Men's Alliance for Medical Marijuana). After spending hours looking through the information there, I was impressed by their mission, their presentation, and their reputation. I took a deep breath and composed an e-mail explaining Jeff's condition in detail and asking for direction.

In all honesty, I was only hoping to be taken seriously. After two anxious days, I received a reply from Valerie Leveroni Corral, WAMM's director, in Santa Cruz, California. She wrote a long and generous note, expressing sympathy for our problem; I believe she sensed my sheer desperation.

Valerie explained that WAMM is a collective of patients, most of them terminally ill, and their caregivers, who all work together to make sure that suffering people can use medical marijuana at no cost. The organization survives solely on donations from members and supporters. As in our case, most severely ill families are stretched to the limit financially. Prescriptions are very expensive. I became an active member of WAMM, even though we lived over a hundred miles away. As members, Jeffrey was able to receive the recommended treatment for free.

Valerie asked me to send all of the documents I had on Jeff, and she put me in touch with a pediatric specialist, Dr. Mike Alcalay, who was experienced with the benefits of using medical marijuana for a variety of ailments. There were no case studies of medical marijuana being used to treat children for mental illness. Dr. Alcalay readily admitted that he didn't know if it would help. In all fairness, this was going to be an experiment as well, the difference being that there were no risks of permanent effects to Jeffrey's overall health. For the first time in a long time, though, I allowed myself some hope.

Jeffrey & WAMM
by Valerie Leveroni Corral

I encountered Debbie and Jeffrey for the first time via email. Debbie had visited our website (www.wamm.org) seeking that proverbial grain of salt from an ocean. We first spoke a few days later, and I was shaken as she unraveled a chilling saga. Jeffrey's aggression, violence and opposition had left her and her family in a near-constant state of stress and dread.

Debbie told me that she had no idea why she had contacted me; it was a shot in the dark.

Her son was facing imminent removal from his school program due to his unmanageability, and would be sent to an institution out of state. She was desperate, and given the gravity of the situation, she was looking for any remaining avenues that might keep her son from being taken from her.

There was only scant evidence to support the use of marijuana in a case such as Jeffrey's, but I thought it should at least be considered a viable option. First I had to review Jeff's records.

What arrived were more than fifty pages of single-spaced, typed documents reflecting the rigorous treatment that Jeff had undergone in a period of only four years. I read and read, fascinated by what lay before me. The medical dossier illustrating Jeffrey's disease, its progression, the procedures and their failures troubled me. I called Debbie and asked her for more information. Her accounts of Jeff's hostility were alarming. It is difficult to witness a mother's despair when her child is suffering, but what could it be like for this kid? My heart broke for this child.

I had observed marijuana's effectiveness on aggressive behavior over the years. Specifically I had seen it work in cases of aggression induced by medications used to treat, among other things, seizures. While Jeffrey was taking no allopathic drugs at the time, it seemed possible that the receptor sites might be encouraged favorably by the use of marijuana.

Part of WAMM's mission has been to keep extensive patient records in order to build documentation of marijuana's specific effects. We use "survey documents" to gather data on marijuana use, its effectiveness on applicable symptoms and to indicate effects marijuana use may have on pharmaceutical use. Two WAMM members with brain dysfunction had shown improvement using marijuana, one child and one adult. It was a long shot, but my own battle with pharmaceutically untreatable epilepsy had convinced me that it was worth a try.

Jeff had been initiated into the world of drugs at age three, experiencing some of the big hitters like Clonodine and Depakote. The side effects of these drugs measured a mountain above anything that marijuana could ever possibly deliver. I felt assured only that we could not cause more harm to Jeffrey.

I helped Debbie connect with Mike Alcalay, MD, a pediatrician who had experience with the therapeutic uses of cannabis. I knew Mike and was aware of the quality and mindful care he provided his patients. He seemed perfect for Jeff's case. Jeff became a member of our collective in May 2001, with his mother acting as his caregiver.

WAMM (Wo/Men's Alliance for Medical Marijuana) is not a buyer's club. We are as much family as anything else. Since we do not buy nor sell marijuana, it is important for each of our members to assume some role in our organization. Completing survey documents or assisting with gardening and administration are some ways that members contribute. An immeasurable benefit our collective provides is the intimacy we develop in building relationships with our members. The relative distance and Jeff's age would preclude him from participation in many of our activities, but each member brings something unique to our group, and Jeff was no exception.

Maternal instinct predisposes a mother to face danger unwittingly, I guess, because I was not afraid of any legal implications. Meanwhile, my parents were watching out the front window for police—they were scared to death about breaking the law, even in light of Proposition 215. But I had read the law's words, and I knew that Jeffrey was protected—he was a Californian who was suffering, and he could possibly benefit from this medication. From where I stood, we had nothing to lose.

I provided WAMM with all of Jeffrey's medical records, IEP's, psychiatric evaluations, and other documents. Dr. Alcalay reviewed every sheet of paper, including Jeff's history and notes from very recent physical examinations, and soon recommended a marijuana regimen.

On May 21, 2001, with nine days left before I would almost certainly lose him, Jeffrey had his first dose of medical marijuana, baked into a muffin provided by WAMM. He was seven and a half years old. In some ways, I've felt like that was the first day of Jeff's life. It came at 8 a.m. that morning, before we made the drive to school. Jeffrey was already dressed when we sat down on the couch and I handed him a quarter of the muffin. He looked at it in the palm of his hand and popped it into his mouth. He didn't seem to mind the taste; it was something new for him and he thought it was cool to be able to eat his medicine—he had taken pills for years. I didn't play it up at all, other than to explain that it was a new medicine and we were going to see if it would help him. He understood that. I held my breath.

As usual, we watched TV before school for a few minutes. I didn't notice anything different about him at all. When it was time to leave, he gave our dog bye-bye kisses and went out the door. He climbed into his car seat in the front passenger side, and as we did every morning, we held hands as I drove. I put the radio on KNCI, his favorite local country station. He loved Pat and Tom, the morning DJ's.

It was a 45-minute trip to his school during rush hour traffic. I merged into the right lane to exit the freeway, and as I entered the city streets, I felt something strange happen between our clasped hands. Jeffrey's grip, always tense and restless, suddenly just loosened. It startled me—usually he clutched my fingers. I glanced over at him, and he was smiling. He said calmly, "Mommy, I feel happy, not mad. And my head doesn't feel noisy." At that moment, the song "I Am Rosemary's Granddaughter," by Jessica Andrews, started playing on the radio. Jeffrey belted out the words, and from then on, it became our song. Within half an hour of ingesting that first piece of muffin, I had a new child. I didn't know whether to keep on driving or pull over and cry.

Medical Marijuana and Children
by Dr. Mike Alcalay

When compared to all other medications, the safety of cannabis is astounding. The measure of a drug's safety is called its therapeutic index, which tells us how many multiples of a medication's effective dose has a potentially lethal effect. The therapeutic index of alcohol and morphine is ten; that is, ten times too much alcohol or morphine becomes the killing dose. For aspirin, Tylenol and ibuprofen it's twenty-five times what is recommended on the package. One hundred times too much penicillin will destroy the kidneys. As for cannabis, there has never been a recorded death from an overdose; in lab animals the dose has been pushed past 40,000 times the recommended one, and the only result is a rat that will curl up in a corner and sleep it off.

Research into the science of marijuana took off in 1964 in the laboratories of Raphael Mechoulam at Jerusalem's Hebrew University. Mechoulam was the first to isolate THC as the primary active ingredient in the plant. But THC is just one of the chemical group of 80 cannabinoids that make up the major medicinal component of the plant. Most cannabinoids are inactive or exist in small amounts; but perhaps up to ten of these appear to produce distinct pharmacological effects in the human body.

Since 1988 research has been skyrocketing. First there was the discovery of receptors on human cells that respond only to cannabinoids. There are two cell receptors types: CB1 receptors in the brain, spinal cord and nerve endings, and CB2 receptors in the immune system, especially the white blood cells and spleen.

Then in 1992, Mecholam's lab isolated a cannabinoid made by our own body, the first of a growing number that are grouped as "endocannabinoids." These endocannabinoids are being found everywhere: at high levels in the blood in brain injury cases and in the birthing process; at lower levels in breast milk, where researchers are postulating that it may play a key role in getting newborns to begin to suckle. A Sanskrit scholar in Mechoulam's lab baptized the first endocannabinoid as anandamide after the Sanskrit word ananda, which means "bliss."

Other interesting research on marijuana's scientific properties and medical applications began during the 1970s, when two

Americans, escaping from government repression in the US landed in cannabis-friendly Amsterdam to begin their scientific studies of the marijuana plant. David Watson and Robert Clarke emerged decades later with not only definitive reference books on cannabis botany and pest management, but carefully bred strains that could yield very specific amounts of very specific cannabinoids.

In time, these strains were transferred to GW Pharmaceutical, a UK-based company run by physician-researcher Geoffrey Guy. Inside a large "secret" greenhouse outside London and under the aegis of the British government, Guy began growing tens of thousands of multiple pure cannabis strains and turning them into various tinctures that are administered as a mouth spray. Next he began performing research study trials, initially on patients with multiple sclerosis, and then on patients with chronic pain from AIDS-related peripheral neuropathy. The results have been very positive and the German-based Bayer pharmaceutical company has picked up the rights to distribute GW's cannabis throughout western Europe, Canada, Australia and New Zealand. US federal law prohibits its distribution in this country.

Their first product is called Sativex and is composed of equal parts sativa and indica. Sativa and indica represent the two poles of the cannabinoid spectrum and the plants generally have their own characteristics and medicinal effects.

Sativas have an effect that tends to be more cerebral. The plant itself grows tall and has light-green long, thin leaves. Indicas have a stronger bodily effect. The indica plant is bushy with dark-green wide leaves. Both sativas and indicas can reduce pain, including migraine headaches, and stimulate the appetite. Sativas have a long list of other uses that include relief from nausea and depression. Sativas tend to increase energy and activity levels, are stimulating and help increase focus and creativity. Indicas, on the other hand, relax the muscles and spasms, for example with MS, reduce the intraocular pressure of glaucoma, act against seizures and work as a sedative for sleep.

Others in the medical profession, most notably, Lester Grinspoon, MD, Harvard professor emeritus, are advocates for the therapeutic properties of cannabis. Dr. Grinspoon has been one of the most outspoken advocates for medical marijuana, especially since seeing the remarkable effects it had on his own young son's treatment for leukemia. When using cannabis, his child went from vomiting incessantly for hours after chemotherapy, to eagerly joining the family for dinner. Similar stories of cannabis use in pediatric patients for chemotherapy are legion and all point to the safety and efficacy of this 5000 year-old Chinese herbal medicine in children.

Chemotherapy has been a common situation in which medical marijuana is recommended, whether for children or adults. Since the passage of Proposition 215, California's medical marijuana initiative, I have seen more than 1200 patients interested in knowing more about medical marijuana. Many of the people I have had the opportunity to spend time with have the typical diagnoses that are associated with marijuana's palliative effects. The rigidity, spasms and pain of multiple sclerosis are visibly relieved as a patient takes a puff or two. Reports of significant decreases in intraocular pressure in glaucoma are overwhelming. And the stimulant effects on the appetite, especially with AIDS patients, are well known. Personally, without medical marijuana I would have succumbed to the wasting syndrome caused by the dysentery of cryptosporidium, which I suffered through several years ago.

Over 99% of the people I have seen were self-medicating with cannabis before I first saw them. Instead of recommending cannabis to people who are already using it, many California physicians are actually approving its continued use. A small but growing number of patients have been self-medicating for both emotional and behavioral diagnoses. After going through the litany of available prescription medications with little or no success, many people that I see are using cannabis for such diagnoses as depression, bipolar disorder, post-traumatic stress disorder, adult attention deficit disorder and Tourette's syndrome. This more controversial use had not yet been suggested in cases of children with behavioral problems.

The proposal to treat Jeffrey's complex diagnosis at his young age with medical marijuana was an unusual scenario from the beginning. My experience with Jeffrey began when Valerie Corral, the co-director of Santa Cruz's WAMM, the Wo/men's Alliance for Medical Marijuana, called in mid-May 2001 and asked if I would talk to a mother who had just contacted her through the WAMM internet site. Val and I have known each other since Proposition 215 passed in California in 1996, and we have a history of talking on the phone on a regular basis about various medical marijuana patients in her group. As Val outlined Jeffrey's case to me, the story she described seemed so outrageous that my first thought was that it must be a setup. In the past few years, several cannabis-prescribing physicians in California have been hassled by both federal and state narcotics officers and the state medical board.

I agreed to speak with Jeffrey's mother Debbie, but with some trepidation. Jeffrey's family lives in the foothills of the Sierras, 2½ hours from my office in Oakland. Debbie and I began our conversation with phone calls and the faxing and mailing of Jeffrey's medical records, and ended with my actually seeing Jeffrey for a physical examination and history.

What first struck me as a pediatrician was this mother's determination to help her child in any way she could and her desperation and fear that her child would soon be taken from her. My review of Jeffrey's medical records and lengthy discussions with the family revealed an emotionally and mentally disturbed 7 year-old child who, in his rather short life, had been evaluated by more than a dozen medical specialists. These physicians had given him a multitude of diagnoses and placed him on a score of heavy-duty prescription medications. All to no avail: Jeffrey was out of control and required 24/7 care and protection.

The dosage I recommended for Jeffrey—one-quarter of a muffin—is one-quarter of WAMM's recommended adult dose. By pharmaceutical standards, it is a very small dose. The PDR's recommendation for Marinol's use in children is to give a full adult dose. Marinol is synthetic THC and is a schedule III drug.

Jeffrey had no untoward effects from taking cannabis. The cannabis mixture that he used had both sativa and indica components. The indica probably helped promote his new sleeping patterns, the sativa his ability to get focused and take on a more pleasant attitude. With the great strides made in cannabinoid research in the past few decades, it is possible we may be dealing with a child who is either deficient in the production of his own endocannabinoids and/or may have defective cannabinoid receptors.

This was our last ditch effort to keep Jeff enrolled at this school and living at home. We had a week to prove it. When we got to school, I took him to his classroom, where I explained to his teacher and counselor that he had started his "new medication" that morning. I had already prepared them for this, and I wanted them to watch him closely and note anything unusual. I almost dropped the note Jeff brought home: "It was wonderful!" his teacher wrote. She reported that he had shown no aggression, and that he had been very compliant and responsive to redirection. Incredibly, Jeff's persona had somehow softened. My parents were almost visibly shaken as they watched him play around the house after school. It was just a day, but nothing had ever happened like this before. He was changed in a profound way—and in a very short time.

From that morning on, Jeff ate a quarter of a muffin twice a day. We were to adjust the dosage according to Dr. Alcalay's well-documented observations. As with any medication, we started out slowly. By now, my mother had embraced the idea of treating Jeff with marijuana. She's always loved to cook, so she asked Valerie for the recipe and began making the muffins at home.

Unfortunately, the muffins weren't a hit with Jeffrey—after the initial novelty of this new method of taking medication wore off, he came to hate the taste. We tried adding the marijuana to brownies and to my mom's best cookie recipes. We even slopped frosting and whipped cream all over our creations, but Jeffrey couldn't stand it. It was Jeffrey himself who came up with the idea of making a pill. My mom researched the Internet and consulted Valerie and Dr. Alcalay, and we came up with a way to cook it while keeping the proper dosage intact.

Transforming the medication from the leaf stage into a capsule was a time-consuming, trial-and-error process. We began by weighing the marijuana, then we put it through a coffee grinder, sifted it, cooked it on the stovetop with butter and water, spread it on a cookie sheet, baked it, cooled it, and then painstakingly filled tiny gelatin capsules with the mixture. Each batch of marijuana was a different color and had a different and often overwhelming smell. Mom turned on every house fan when she was cooking it. I never got used to the strong odor myself, but I never felt any effects from breathing it in. The smell alone didn't alter us in any way.

The process took over five hours. The capsules were produced in two different sized gelatin capsules, which made it easier to adjust the dosage. The method became much more efficient when our local health food store manager told me about a machine called a "pill packer." I ordered it right away and my mom soon became known around the house as the "Pill Packin' Grandma," with great affection. We did find that by the end of a month's supply, the medicine wasn't as effective. Valerie suggested we make smaller batches for two to three weeks at a time. It was more work, but it solved the problem. Jeff got one large and one small capsule each morning and evening, and one large capsule at 1:30 p.m.

For each batch we received, we had to take a wait-and-see approach. Different formulas had different effects and we had to wait to finally arrive at a combination that worked best for Jeff. In the beginning, we could tell within a few hours how a certain recipe had affected him—we could literally see him calm down. One combination of strains had too strong an effect—it made him giddy and very lovey-dovey—full of hugs and pet names for us. We didn't use that mixture again.

The chemistry of marijuana was a mystery to me. Then again, so was every other pill Jeffrey had taken. I knew nothing about the varieties of marijuana or how Jeffrey's formula was determined. Valerie kept meticulous records—she knows her subject well—but we didn't know if it was the grade or the quality or the variety that made the difference. We weren't aware of what Valerie had to "tweak" to improve the mix. When she arrived at the correct formulation, it was obvious.

In order to keep things simple, we told Jeffrey that his medicine was called "amino acids." We didn't want him to be teased at school, or for any parents to be alarmed if he happened to tell his peers that he was taking marijuana. Every time Jeff came into the house while Mom was preparing his batch, he'd say, "Smells like amino acids in here!" Sometimes we'd walk by a doorway or someone on the street and Jeff would happily declare, "He smells like amino acids!"

Chapter 9

SIX MONTHS LATER, MY eight year-old son wasn't angry with the world. He was actually learning how to have fun, and, for the first time ever, his outbursts had diminished enough so that he was capable of benefiting from psychological and behavioral counseling. For Jeff's eighth birthday, he invited a dozen friends to a party at a pizza place. He had been stable enough to go out to restaurants with us in the past few months, and if anyone deserved some fun, it was Jeff. We were delighted when all of Jeff's invited guests showed up, gifts in hand. It was the first time we'd been able to throw a celebration for Jeff, and there wasn't a single problem that afternoon. Seeing Jeffrey experience something most children take for granted was miraculous. That winter, neighborhood kids who hadn't been allowed to play with Jeffrey were knocking on our door to see if he could come out and ride his bike or skate.

Jeff was able to maintain control almost all the time. In general, he was treating everyone kindly, including our new dog, a mini-Schnauzer called Jaspur who would become Jeffrey's constant playmate and "baby brother." A friend gave us a fish tank about two months after he started the medication. Jeffrey and I went to the pet store and bought a neon tetra, a couple of guppies, and a snail. Against my better judgment, I let Jeff talk me into keeping the tank in his bedroom. I instructed him never, ever to feed the fish. I was afraid he would dump the entire bottle of food in the water and kill them. In all honesty, I expected to find the creatures dead the next morning. Not only were they still living, but they had also reproduced! My first reaction was panic, but Jeff was delighted by what he called the little "eyeballs" in the tank. We giggled ourselves silly trying to count how many new babies there were. This was more like what I had expected from motherhood. This was the mother/son relationship I had dreamed of.

When Jeffrey had come home from residential care in February 2001, he'd been overweight—a side effect of all the medications. He was 46 inches tall and weighed 86 pounds. Now, he was 48 inches tall and weighed 65 pounds. Contrary to the common belief that marijuana increases appetite, Jeffrey actually ate less. The change in Jeffrey was phenomenal. He had more energy and he was enjoying himself.

The positive effects of the marijuana on Jeffrey's behavior were too profound to be questioned. Still, proof of how much the medicine was helping him came when Jeff had to have his tonsils removed. We stopped giving him marijuana just prior to surgery. He came out of the operation in a physically and verbally assaultive and agitated state; the more pain medication he was given, the more violent he became, and his tolerance for pain was very low. His obsessive-compulsive disorders resurfaced within hours. Jeff woke up from the surgery in a rage, angry at everyone and everything. He couldn't scream, because his throat was raw, but he made plenty of noise by throwing anything he could get his hands on. He wouldn't accept any comfort whatsoever. This continued for a couple of days until he decided his throat was well enough to swallow his "amino acids." Within an hour, he had calmed down.

Medical marijuana was not a cure. We recognized that Jeff had underlying problems that needed to be addressed. Unlike previous treatments, medical marijuana allowed Jeff to participate in therapy, go to school, live at home, and have friends. He seemed like a typical kid, and he was beginning to develop social skills, which his behavioral problems had prevented before now. When we'd been given 30 days to come up with a solution we'd been searching for over many years, we had considered our odds to be very bad. But the school recognized Jeff's progress. The countdown to expulsion—and an inevitable move out of state—had almost miraculously come to an end. Not only was Jeff able to stay in his current program, but we were getting very few calls and notes sent home about bad behavior. The county even expected to be able to mainstream him into public school within the next year or two. We were living a different life—we went shopping and skating. Jeffrey and I enjoyed bowling together. After the whirlwind of doctors and pills, we had finally found something that helped.

Medical marijuana was a blessing, but it wasn't an absolute miracle. We knew that there were never any guarantees. Life was not perfect. Jeffrey was still angry and defiant at times, and he continued to lack some social skills—but these issues were all being addressed now, and we could finally see some real progress. All we could do was hope and pray that the medical marijuana would continue to help him. It seemed to all of us that Jeff was learning how to really think about his problems for the first time. He was becoming introspective.

Jeffrey and I have always had a little personal saying: "Love your guts." Jeff knows that no matter what, no matter how "icky" things might get, I will always love him. When I heard Jeff say that he felt "happy and not mad," it had been a monumental step forward. We still had challenges before us. It was a case of one step at a time. But now we knew that he could manage his problems enough to enjoy a more regular life.

～

From the beginning of our exploration into medical marijuana, I had insisted that everything be done legally and ethically. Especially after I'd put my faith in this treatment, I wanted to be completely honest with everyone involved in Jeffrey's life. We didn't make a point of telling people outright, but if asked, we were always truthful. During my research phase, almost everyone had been supportive; some people had been doubtful that marijuana would help, but no one had suggested that we abandon the idea. Our social circle was mainly fellow church members, and many had lived through the heartache with us from the time Jeff was a toddler. Even our pastor expressed support. Although he was neutral and non-committal, he told us he thought it was a brave and loving thing to do. When medical marijuana showed positive effects, everyone was delighted. The improvement in Jeffrey's behavior said it all.

My parents had initially been nervous about informing the county and Jeff's counselors and social workers about his new treatment. After the fact, though, they were relieved that I had chosen to share the information. It added credibility to both my research and my decision, and it also demonstrated my insistence on following the letter of the law. Ironically, despite all of my good intentions, a battle was festering.

Jeffrey had been using the new medication for a month and a half, and things were going better than we'd ever imagined. There were no warning signs leading up to the phone call I received in late June informing me of a "change in my court date." Court date? I had no idea what the clerk was talking about. According to the limited information I could gather, a report had been made to Child Protective Services (CPS), accusing me of being an unfit mother and of contributing to the delinquency of a minor. We were completely blindsided by the order that we were to appear before the court on charges of child endangerment.

Mom and I worked frantically all weekend preparing paperwork for the judge, and I spent hours on the phone trying to solicit help and advice regarding some plan of action. I called Dr. Alcalay first, and he referred me to Bill Panzer, an attorney who had participated in the creation of Proposition 215. Mr. Panzer referred me to Wendell Peters, a local attorney.

From what I understood, two things were at stake in this case: Jeffrey could potentially be taken away from me, and he would have to go off of this very successful medication. Anger eclipsed all my other emotions. After everything we had been through, after being upfront with all parties, and after finally finding something that worked, I was being officially and publicly accused of hurting my son. The thought of going back to where we'd been before was chilling.

I already knew that under California's Proposition 215, it was legal to give medical marijuana to a severely ill patient. Many agreed that Jeff qualified. Our friends, family, doctors, and Jeff's teachers had seen first-hand how marijuana had positively affected him. What I didn't realize was that although Jeff had a doctor's recommendation, it was not recognized by the federal government. This was incredibly confusing to me. In retrospect, I had no idea that the federal government could overrule my doctor's opinion and my state's law. I am a mother first, a Californian second, and a U.S. citizen last. I felt violated to the core.

I had angels on my side, though. Glen Backes at the Lindesmith Center arranged for legal representation to be provided by the Drug Policy Alliance and the California chapter of the National Organization for the Reform of Marijuana Laws (NORML), through the Medical Marijuana Patients' and Caregivers' Fund. Created in 1994, the Lindesmith Center is an organization whose mission is to inform the public debate on drug policy and related issues. It is one of the leading independent drug policy organizations in the United

States. California NORML is a non-profit, membership-supported organization dedicated to educating and encouraging people to reconsider and legalize marijuana through the publication of a newsletter, sponsoring scientific research, lobbying lawmakers, hosting events, and offering legal, educational, and consumer health advice. Together, these two invaluable resources handled all of the legal aspects of the court case, including retaining Mr. Peters as my attorney. Amazingly, everyone simply told me not to worry about the cost—that it would be taken care of. It was a Godsend as I had no money to defend myself and my son.

The trial started on July 3, 2001, only one week after we'd received the ominous phone call. The first court date was very frightening. It appeared that county services had one goal in mind: for Jeffrey to be removed from the medication immediately. Mr. Peters wasn't even in town. He'd been given little time to prepare, and he had a conflicting court date with another client on the east coast. He was forced to "appear" in court via telephone. My parents and a close friend went with me; they were asked to identify themselves and explain why they were there. The judge thanked them for their time and support. The reception we received was, I am confident, out of the norm; then again, we were not the typical family they saw day in and day out appearing in a drug or child endangerment case.

Jeffrey did not attend any of the court appearances. Fitting in had always been an issue with him, and if he'd felt like his "amino acids" were a bad thing, it would have devastated him.

We handed over the extensive background reports detailing all of Jeffrey's medical, behavioral, and educational histories to the judge, and he called a three-hour recess to examine them. When we reconvened, the judge declared Jeffrey to be a "medical experiment." He ordered that Jeffrey "stay put" until further investigation into additional evaluation and medication alternatives could be conducted by the prosecuting team. In other words, we left the court with the judge's approval to keep Jeffrey at home, continuing his medicine. Now, someone else would have to look for alternative treatments. It seemed like good news, all things considered.

The second court date was two weeks later, but no additional information had been collected by the prosecuting team. The "stay put" order remained in effect. This time, paper was taped over the courtroom windows, and we were shuffled in and out through the back door into an alley in order to escape the media who had gathered outside. The judge issued a gag order, and reporters were barred from the proceedings. As long as the media protected Jeffrey's privacy, we were okay with the coverage this case was sure to bring. We also looked at it as an opportunity to alert other parents to the possibility that there was hope and help for their own out-of-control children. The average pediatrician, therapist, and psychiatrist certainly weren't sharing much information about the potential benefits of medical marijuana.

On July 11, 2001, an article appeared on the front page of our local newspaper: "Medical Pot War Engulfs Boy, 7—Mom Says Cannabis Muffins Aid His Brain Disorder." The article was received by readers in a generally positive way, and supportive feedback poured in from the community. I found the media in general to be unbiased and their reporting based on fact. In truth, many reporters listened and responded to us better than most of Jeffrey's doctors had!

Over the next four months, there were several more court dates, but the prosecution team was never able to come up with any definite alternative treatment or plan. Arrangements were made for Jeffrey to be examined by a doctor from the University of California at Davis. It was to be a non-biased examination, but when he presented his report in court, it was sorely one-sided: the doctor said that the medications Jeffrey had received in the past had not failed, but that, "the mother had...in not giving (them) to him as 'enthusiastically' as she had the medical marijuana." The court recognized the bias. Much of Jeff's medication had been administered by doctors in his residential care facilities. Had they lacked enthusiasm as well?

In the end, I think the judge, as well as the county, just wanted the messy situation to go away. The subject was inflammatory, and we were caught up in a political knot of conflicting ideas about marijuana. On the one hand, giving marijuana to a child was among the most controversial applications of Proposition 215—it easily pushed the panic button for skeptics of marijuana's legitimacy as a medicine. On the other hand, there was the heartbreak of a suffering little boy and his desperate family. In the end, the extensive documentation of Jeffrey's history protected us.

Because Jeffrey's history was well documented, everyone involved could see that there was no recklessness on my part. A wide variety of sources testified that Jeffrey was doing much better. Our case was wasting court time and money. On December 4, 2001, the case was dismissed. The only stipulation was that Jeffrey would be required to see a pediatrician every six months for testing and evaluation. It was a landmark ruling as there had been no previous cases of medical marijuana being recommended for children with severe mental/behavioral problems. The judge expressed sympathy for all that our family had been through and wished us success. On December 5, 2001, our local paper's headline read: "Mom Keeps Son On Marijuana Regimen." Again, the response was very positive.

Of course, I was primarily relieved; but I also held a lingering anger that we had been forced to go to court in the first place. It was terribly ironic that I had voted against Proposition 215. Thank goodness other people had been more educated than I was at the time. Otherwise, my son would have been in an institution by now.

In July, the CBS television newsmagazine 48 HOURS contacted me and requested an interview after learning about the court case in the newspaper. We were naturally concerned about Jeff's, and the family's, privacy. As grateful as we were for medical marijuana, the last thing we wanted was for Jeff to become a nationally recognized poster child. All he ever wanted was to be "normal." The program's producer assured us that we could maintain our anonymity, and that Jeff would be filmed in a way that would protect him from being easily identified. I had no fear of appearing on camera. Although I didn't want my full name to be mentioned, I believed strongly that I could help other families by sharing our experiences. After much discussion, we decided to allow a team to fly in from New York—a producer, an interviewer (Harold Dow), two cameramen, and a soundman—to tape Jeffrey and our family, our daily routine, and to conduct interviews with Dr. Alcalay. The goal was to capture a typical day in our lives. Jeff and our family were filmed interacting together. They showed my mom and I preparing his medication, and they spoke to me at length. Furniture was rearranged, cameras were placed at both ends of our living room and kitchen, huge umbrellas were set up to reflect light, and microphones were wired inside our clothing. It felt like a mammoth production, though Jeffrey weathered it with calm. With all the social workers in and out of the house, he was already used to a crowd. The experience was a pleasure—everyone involved was kind, easy to talk to, and nonjudgmental. I do believe they were somewhat surprised that our family was so "typical"—I'm not sure what they expected at first. In time, they even shared our excitement that medical marijuana had made such a huge difference in Jeff's life.

In all, the crew made three separate visits over a period of several months. Six hours of film were reduced to an eight-minute segment by the time the show aired. The program's theme addressed the validity of four different situations, one of which was: "Should this mother be allowed to give her seven year old son medical marijuana?" It aired on March 6, 2002, after the court case had been dismissed, and received remarkably positive viewer feedback. Eighty-eight percent of viewers who called in to voice their opinion voted that, "Yes, she should be allowed to provide her ill son with medical marijuana."

The morning after the show aired, I was standing in a coffee shop when a woman looked at me very intensely and approached me. "Aren't you the mom from TV last night?" she asked. Before I could answer, she hugged me. "I saw the preview for the program and I called my friend right away. Neither of us believed that marijuana had any medicinal value until we saw your story." For a full five minutes, she kept repeating, "What a mom, what a mom. Thank you for being so strong and brave." I was taken aback, but this was just the first of many such occurrences. People recognized me everywhere I went. Over the next weeks, we received phone calls from all over the country from parents who had out-of-control children and were desperately afraid of losing them to the system. I remembered so well when I'd felt all alone, watching reports on television about children like Jeff. I did my best to listen and to offer sympathy, but I redirected most calls to WAMM. They were the experts, after all. We also received a multitude of e-mail; people wanted more information. I was eager to share—I had walked in those shoes, and I knew the heartache. I knew that medical marijuana was not a "fix-all" for every troubled child, but I also felt that everyone deserved access to reliable information, at the very least.

From: ▓▓▓▓▓▓▓▓▓▓▓▓▓
Sent: Thursday, March 07, 2002 12:01 AM
To: CND 48Hours
Subject: Recipe for Trouble

How can I get more info about his situation? This is a mirror of what is happening with my 9 year old son. We don't know what to do.

From: ▓▓▓▓▓▓▓▓▓▓▓▓▓
Sent: Wednesday, March 06, 2002 10:58 PM
To: Debbie
Subject: Marijuana and your son

I have a son who has ADHD and is oppositional defiant as well. I was very moved by your story and am happy you found success in helping your son. We have gone through a great deal of heartache with our son also. He is the youngest of five children and different. Can you let me know who the doctor is who prescribed the marijuana for you? I would also like to know how you prepare this medication for your son as I am interested in exploring this alternative for my son. Thanking you in advance.

From: ▓▓▓▓▓▓▓▓▓▓▓▓
Sent: Thursday, March 07, 2002 9:16 AM
To: Debbie
Subject: 48 hours story

Hi Debbie,
I have to tell you that your story really gave me hope. My son has almost the same diagnosis as your son. He has ADHD, bi-polar disorder (with psychotic features) and ODD as well as behavioral problems. He has been on many of the same medications as your son as well. He is 10 years old. We are really struggling with aggression problems, and the mood swings. Medication helps lessen the severity, but does not control the mood changes like it should. I am very interested to talk with you about your experi-

ence. Where did you find the doctor? Is it possible to contact him? I live in Salt Lake City, Utah, and am not even sure that prescription marijuana is available here. I would definitely like to hear more about it. He is on four different kinds of medication right now, and it is a lot of pills with not a great result. Any information or advice you could give me would be greatly appreciated.

From: ▮▮▮▮▮▮▮▮▮▮▮▮▮▮
Sent: Wednesday, March 06, 2002 6:28 PM
TO: 48hours
Subject: show aired on March 6, 2002, CA

How do we go about contacting your guest on the topic of her child who has the behavioral disorders? I have the same problem and would like further information on the difference the marijuana made. My child is 10 years old and has been diagnosed with Tourette's Syndrome, ODD, ADD, and OCD. He is currently on four different drugs and still is out of control, and I give him one drug around the clock every four hours. If you can forward this email to the mom maybe she can email me back with more information.

From: ▮▮▮▮▮▮▮▮▮▮▮▮▮
Sent: Thursday, March 07, 2002 7:49 AM
To: Debbie
Subject: hello Debbie
I got your email from the gal at 48 hours and wanted to let you know I support you 100%. We also have a child who sounds just like yours...she has been on all the same drugs as your son and has been under a doctor's care since age 3. We would love to try the medicine that helped your son. Does it have a name? Would it be possible to know what the drug is and the strength? Perhaps I could ask the doctor if he would try it for her? Thanks for your help!!

From: ■■■■■■■■■■■■■■■
Sent: Wednesday, March 06, 2002 7:47 PM
To: Debbie
Subject: Your 48 hours show
Hello Ms. Jeffries:

I have never been so moved as to write a letter to a perfect
stranger as I was after watching the special on 48 hours. I cried
through it while my husband had to leave the room. I am in NC
and lost my son to our local Social Services four years ago when
he was 12 years old because I walked the same path as you...10+
doctors, multiple diagnosis including ADHD, OCD, Tourettes,
ODD, to name but a few...every medication known to mankind,
3 inpatients hospitalizations, 2 6-month residential stays...all
this at the recommendation of the drs. One day I lost my temper
and made a fatal mistake. He called me a foul name and, having never heard it from him before and being a Christian who
does not partake in such language, smacked him on the mouth...
it was a knee-jerk reaction but enough to warrant an investigation. During which, the very frustrated Drs. (frustrated with me
AND their lack of effectiveness) actually recommended that he
be placed in a group home where he can not hurt anyone until
he is 18. Yes, they threw my child away and the charges against
us were Inappropriate Discipline and Neglect. That was 4 years
ago...so what I'd like to say to you is: Congratulations...stay the
course. You are a great mother and are doing a wonderful thing
for your son. Whatever your faith, know that you and your son
will always be in my prayers. I only wish I had had access to this
information years ago and perhaps my son would be allowed to
grow up with his older sister and younger brother and his two
parents who love him beyond measure.

From: ████████████████████
Sent: Thursday, March 07, 2002 12:45 AM
To: DND 48 Hours
Subject: 8 year old on medical marijuana

I think this Mom was really dedicated to her son. I too, am in this position. My son is almost a mirror image of this boy only he is 13 1/2 years old and currently is taking both Seroquel and Adderall. He had been given a resent increase in Seroquel and his whole body turned green! His face, arms, hands, elbows, even his blood vessels were green tinted. He was rushed to the Drs. When I called to ask about his color. After several Drs. and nurses were all stunned and blood tests revealed nothing his meds were reduced again and he returned to normal.

He has temper out bursts, dangerous episodes (no clear thinking) i.e. talking to strangers, straying away from home, hearing voices, attacking pregnant mom on more than one occasion, hitting people—day care workers and students (no daycare wanted him or could handle him), I was charged/accused with child abuse 3-4 times (all eventually dismissed), smearing of feces, seeing dead people (they talk to him—the devil), failing school, lock up in mental institution, special schools, special ed, treatment centers, etc.

I would love to try this on my son. In Colorado though medical marijuana is not accepted even though voters once passed this issue…I do not want to see my son on drugs (which he is against) but look at the powerful drugs he is on now!!! We have tried them all, and of course with different side effects!! One of the worst medications made him twitch and wet the bed. He sits with his mouth open sometimes, which reminds me of a zombie or a medical patient in a ward heavily sedated.

I really feel for Debbie and I certainly understand her reasoning. Do you know how I can reach her? Are there places (hospitals, Drs.) in Colorado that could or would prescribe this? This is one of the stories that the medical profession needs to hear/see and also the legislatures/system regulators should take note. This has to be less addictive and less expensive than these other medications with less side effects, what munchies?

Do you have anything else on this story or the Doctor involved for my research?

Chapter 10

WHILE JEFF HAD BEEN living in residential placement, I met a wonderful man. I married Bob in March 2002. Despite the many complications and difficulties of my family life, our relationship became a source of love, security, and comfort for me. I had waited several months before introducing Jeffrey to him, but Bob knew everything there was to know about Jeff and his problems. Bob's compassion for my son was one of the many things about him I fell in love with. By the time they met, I had already begun researching medical marijuana, and Bob agreed that it was a sound idea. A year later, Jeffrey was eight years old; he was responding positively to the new medicine; he was successfully attending school, and he was living at home on our wedding day.

In Spring of that year, Jeff had a daddy, and I firmly believed that having a strong father figure around was excellent therapy for him. Jeff also had a new 14-year-old brother and 12-year-old sister. Before Bob proposed to me, he had spoken to his kids at length about Jeff's situation. Mark and Brittney met Jeffrey for the first time after he'd begun the medical marijuana therapy, and they had never witnessed any of his extreme behavior. My new stepchildren realized that Jeff had issues, but they felt like they could handle it.

Actually living with Jeff, though, turned out to be more trying than anyone had bargained for. They did their best to accept him, but no teenagers really want to hang out with an eight-year-old little brother, anyway. There were true moments of tenderness between Jeff and Brittney; Mark, on the other hand, promised not to "kill" Jeff, and we all thought that was as close as we were going to get.

With my new marriage came a new home in another county in central California. Bob's kids were well established in their schools, and moving them would have been unfair and possibly even detrimental to their educational and social progress. We were ready to try anything to create a happy family with as little upheaval as possible. Fortunately, Jeff adjusted well to his new classroom in a special day class for SED children in a regular public school. We knew this was only possible through his continued use of medical marijuana.

It wasn't long before we ran into some serious problems, however. The IEP from our former county was already in place, and it had been agreed upon that Jeff's services would be transferred and maintained, along with his marijuana treatment. This included one-on-one therapy and community therapy—which consisted of a counselor taking Jeff on outings to places like the mall, skate parks, and the bowling alley. This provided a much needed weekly respite for the family as well as maintaining an effort to improve Jeff's social skills. Although the new county had initially agreed to accept Jeff's old IEP, we were soon informed that such services were basically non-existent there. The new county's attitude seemed to be that as long as a student was able to receive an education (even if the child had to be massively medicated), the school was performing its due diligence. There was no arguing the point—they were adamant about their position and offered no compromise whatsoever.

To complicate things even more, we were told that Jeff would not be able to take his "meds" on school grounds. This county was already aware of the court's decision, but a mental health intake worker at the county office opined one day that I had somehow "gotten away" with something by treating Jeffrey with marijuana. She insisted that there was little they would do to accommodate his needs. This is no exaggeration—the difference between the support provided by the two different counties was like night and day. They blamed their unwillingness to transfer his services on a lack of funding, saying that they had been advised by their own attorneys–even though medical marijuana was legal in the state, it was illegal federally. The local school district would be in danger of losing their federal funding if his meds were administered on campus. So, Jeff rode the education transportation van every morning to school, and at lunchtime I would drive to his school to give Jeff his capsule. After I arrived, I would have to check Jeff out so that I could administer his medication to him off school grounds. Jeff thought this was as silly as I did since he knew other students were given their medicine right there at school by the nurse or teachers. He did say that he hated the fact that they were "forcing him to be different."

These new developments made things inconvenient, but not impossible. I was a full-time mom while Bob worked, so I was able to spend the necessary time driving back and forth to his school. Then Bob lost his job. After searching for four months, he still wasn't able to find a new position, even out of his field. I took a job for a construction company

On the positive side, Bob was able to get Jeff up in the morning and have some alone time with him; they played pool, rode skateboards in the driveway, played basketball, and ate breakfast together. The special-ed van continued to pick Jeffrey up each morning and return him home each afternoon; Bob would take care of him until I returned home. When Bob found work again, Jeff was dropped off at an after-school Boy's Club program.

While the marijuana was helping enormously, there were still incidents, though they were less frequent and less intense. Between a new school and a new family, new problems were bound to surface. Jeffrey loved his brother and sister, but adjustments needed to be made on everyone's part. When we took a family vacation to Mexico, Mark and Brittney faced the realities of being with Jeff on a full-time basis for the first time. Within a few days, Jeff had a number of mishaps—he lost his goggles and wanted another pair, but then he lost those, too. He argued about where he was going to sleep, what he was going to wear, and what to watch on TV. In under a week, the whole family was on edge. This was the first time we had all been together with no breaks from Jeff, and we were there for two weeks—Grandma and Grandpa had stayed at home. We were forced to return early—it was just too much. Mark and Brittney forgave Jeff, but they also vowed never, ever to go on a family vacation again. I couldn't really blame them.

All things considered, though, 2002 had been a step in the right direction for us. Jeffrey and I finished our bowling league, he had been able to spend hours at the skate park without altercations with other children, he was performing well in school, and he had participated in Boy's Club activities every day with no problems. He wasn't receiving the therapy and psychiatric care our former county had provided, and he wasn't experiencing any monumental headway in recovery, but neither was he regressing. There was still hope for a better future for Jeffrey. He continued to take his "amino acids" and attend group therapy at his school until late summer. That's when the state and the federal government's battle over medical marijuana took a turn that would change our lives as it did the lives of many Proposition 215 patients and their families throughout California.

On September 6, 2002, a television producer I had befriended called to ask me what I thought of the big news. He was sure I had already heard about it and wanted to make sure we were okay. On that day, the national news had reported about a DEA raid on WAMM in Santa Cruz, where 250 members had been working collectively to grow medicine for benefit of the ill. The crop was destroyed; arrests were made.

My immediate reaction was tears. That soon turned to fear. Were we a target? Would they come after us next? After being on *48 Hours,* the federal government surely knew where we lived. I felt profound anguish for Valerie and WAMM, along with all of the people I knew were going to suffer—including Jeffrey. How could this have happened? We lived in California, and our state's citizens had passed Proposition 215. We had a legal right to use marijuana recommended by a doctor for medicinal purposes. How could these rights be ignored? How could votes be deemed worthless? WAMM was the farm where we all got our free and legal medication, and now we had lost our only source of aid.

With his medication abruptly halted, Jeffrey began a new downhill slide almost immediately, and we were thrown right back into a period of uncertainty. As I have learned throughout this experience, medicinal marijuana is a very complex subject. Not only is the individual dosage important, but the qualities of the plant make all the difference. Plants with different ratios of cannabinoids, the active ingredients, have different medical effects. Valerie and Dr. Alcalay had worked tirelessly to determine which and how much of a particular blend of plants Jeffrey responded to. When Jeffrey's formulation had been created, it was completely unique—a tremendous amount of work had gone into it. But with the raid, all of this hard work was lost—it had been taken by the DEA.

During the month of September, we were only able to acquire an inferior quality of marijuana that had been donated. It did not look the same, smell the same, or have the same positive results.

Jeffrey's aggression increased; the physical fights started again, and he had problems at school. It wasn't long before we could no longer eat dinner together as a family because mealtime had become such an ordeal; the teens served themselves and went their separate ways and Bob and I tried to sit with Jeff for as long as we all could. Mark and Brittney needed our attention, too; but most of our time had to be spent dealing with Jeffrey. As I watched Jeffrey regress, I was filled with despair—for myself, for my family, and for my son. And I was furious with my government.

Because the IEP services Jeffrey had been receiving before we moved had been eliminated, we were referred to a therapist through our local HMO. After reading through Jeffrey's history, he said, "Well, why don't you just let him break everything in his room if he is angry? Just let him break his own stuff, not yours." He made this statement in front of Jeffrey. We never returned to his office.

Jeff's mental health was deteriorating rapidly. November brought more physical fights, more calls to pick him up at school, more trouble with authority, and more serious problems at home. He had to be on "line-of-sight" supervision by an adult at all times. At the end of the month, he was banned from the Boy's Club after beating an older and bigger boy who had been taunting him. Jeff was small, but fearless, and his physical attacks instilled terror in both the other boys and the staff there.

Soon, Jeff's violence was drawing other, even more ominous, attention. In the past few weeks, two law enforcement officers, on two different occasions, had come to our home after we'd been forced to use take-down techniques to subdue him. In full uniform, including their side arms, they spoke with Jeffrey about "going down the wrong road." They explained, with dead seriousness, that at his age there wasn't much they could do—but once he was 12 years old, his behavior would land him in "lock up" at the California Youth Authority. It didn't phase Jeff, but it sure did scare us. I couldn't help but wonder what was going to become of Jeffrey as a man if this aggression couldn't be solved. What kind of man would Jeffrey be, and what effect would he have on the world around him? What horrendous situations were ahead of us still? Twelve was less than three years away.

Everything from the past that we had agonized over was rearing its ugly head all over without Jeffrey's medicine. We had been so hopeful that we would never again have to live in constant fear of what he was going to do, who he was going to hurt, or how he would react in any situation. But now the old behavior was back in full force. He gained 20 pounds in a matter of months, and this extra weight added fuel to his constant state of rage as well as increasing his amazing strength during his violent episodes. One night, out of the blue, Jeffrey did something he hadn't done in a long while. After I refused to let him stay up past his bedtime to watch a WWF wrestling match on TV, he grabbed a fork and threatened to stab me to death.

My sense of overwhelming defeat was combined with rage. Our federal government's misguided marijuana policy was causing my ill child to suffer. It seemed obvious to me, at least, that real criminals should be the target—not sick people using safe and seemingly legal medical treatments. I cried because I didn't understand how I could live in the United States, the "Land of the Free," and yet my son's only chance for real freedom against fear, toxic medication, and the harsh reality of being shackled to a hospital bed in a mental ward had been swept away. All of WAMM's work had been confiscated, and I was utterly powerless. Who was being hurt? What were we being protected from? No one was even making any money!

Things simply could not continue under these conditions, but we were at a loss as to where to turn. Residential care began to look like a certainty. We continued trying to recreate the perfect combination, variety, and dosage in Jeff's treatment with the aid of Dr. Alcalay and WAMM, as well as developing a comprehensive therapy plan. Jeffrey would soon be ten years old, and many doctors had insisted that after a certain age, beginning around puberty, the window of opportunity to treat a child's underlying problems would slam shut. We were running out of time.

No formal charges were filed following the raid, and WAMM resumed operations, but without their crop, their task was like a desperate case of triage as they tried to meet the immediate needs of many of their members. At Valerie and Dr. Alcalay's suggestion, we agreed to stop all medical marijuana for the month of December 2002 while they searched for adequate plants to make a new formulation. This made sense to me because it was the same protocol we had followed with all of Jeffrey's past medications. December was grueling. Jeffrey told me, "I wish my medicine worked, because I can make better decisions and I'm not so bad when I take it."

We had been trying unsuccessfully to solicit the help of a county-appointed psychiatrist since we'd moved to this new county nine months prior. The whole family needed psychiatric guidance by this time. During that long month of December, we were able to get an appointment with the county mental health psychiatrist. We approached it with guarded anticipation: now that Jeffrey was a little older, maybe one of the prior medications would treat him more successfully. Perhaps he would be able to assess Jeffrey's current condition and make some recommendations. We just wanted a glimmer of hope.

The appointment started off in a promising way, because it was clear the doctor had taken the time to read over Jeffrey's entire file, including his pharmaceutical history. As we discussed the fact that he had lost his medical marijuana and had regressed to his old behavior problems, the doctor looked at me and said, "Well, I have seen many kids. There is, unfortunately, not much hope for kids like Jeff. He is headed down the wrong path and eventually he will be in trouble with the law."

Amazed, I retorted, "That is why we are here, to try to prevent that and head him down the right road!"

He lowered his gaze and gave me a sad smile. "You cannot treat oppositional defiance," he said. I insisted that something had to be done because our family was in turmoil. "Maybe we should medicate the family instead!" he answered, as if he thought I'd find his response humorous. I pressed on. I questioned him about the availability of any help for families in need in the county. He stressed that there was nothing further he could offer. He was very clear. Then he said he didn't see a need to make another appointment. I wondered if I'd heard him correctly. I had hit a brick wall—there were no more avenues of help.

Chapter 11

ON THE LAST DAY of 2002, we had the new marijuana formula. We crossed our fingers, hoping that it would bring relief. An hour later, we asked Jeff how he felt—whether he could tell that he'd taken his new medication. He thought for a second and said, "Yes. I don't feel so mad. I feel better."

Over the next couple of weeks, the dynamics again began to change within our family to a certain degree. Jeff's constant attention-seeking and aggressive acting-out diminished. We were able to spend more time with Mark and Brittney, and everyone was getting along better. We enrolled Jeff in an after-school program at our neighborhood elementary school. He was allowed to go to the skate park and we didn't fear the worst. He was regaining privileges with his positive behavior and attitude.

We waited and watched while Jeff had good days and bad days, good hours and bad hours. The positive effects of the new formula lasted less than a month, though. While he'd still had some small behavioral setbacks during his treatment, Jeff's violence, specifically, had been appeased with the original medical marijuana recipe. Now, the negative behavior was on the rise, but it was also accompanied by violence. Valerie and Dr. Alcalay adjusted the formula again, but Jeff began exhibiting the physical outbursts—kicking, punching, and biting—that had been among the most disturbing of his previous symptoms.

In the next months, new formulas were experimented with

again and again. We held onto a fragile strand of hope because we knew from experience that medical marijuana could have a tremendously positive impact on Jeff's behavior. It had a proven track record as far as we were concerned. But it just didn't happen. By summer, Jeff was completely out of control, and when school started in the fall, it was only a few days before we knew he'd be forced to leave. No after-school program would accept him.

Since the doctors had told us that we had to find help for Jeffrey before the age of 12 or 13, we could practically hear the seconds ticking away. Medication, parenting, counseling, and therapeutic components could help to effect this change—but there also had to be a certain level of maturity so that he could grasp and respond to all those forces. To me, that seemed contradictory. Jeff needed to grow emotionally and intellectually in order to benefit from therapy; on the other hand, the "experts" had proclaimed that after a certain age, he would be a "lost cause."

I clearly recognized that medical marijuana had given Jeff the ability to think things through more, to consider options and make weighed decisions. It had allowed him periods of normalcy—something no other medication had accomplished. But beneath it all, there was a serious problem that needed to be resolved. Our ultimate hope had always been that the use of this medication would open Jeff up to participating in the therapy he needed—that it would act as a bridge of sorts. Valerie never stopped trying to recreate that certain blend that Jeffrey had responded so well to; she did the best she could with what she'd been left with. When we realized the formula couldn't be recreated, as any pharmaceutical medication could have been; when it didn't make a dynamic positive difference in Jeffrey, I opted to stop it altogether. The decision was heartbreaking. We had reached a point where Jeffrey's behavior had become too much for us to manage. My parents were still strong, but they were older. Jeffrey was bigger, and with his strength, the damage he was able to inflict was very daunting. Now, it was even a possibility that Jeffrey would soon do something that would land him in trouble with the law. If we didn't find help, he could eventually be lost to the prison system. He was also more dangerous to himself than he'd ever been. We were faced with the possibility of a residential program, a psychiatric hospital, or an out-of-state Level 14 facility. Instead, we decided to find a place that would be safe, compassionate, and willing to accept him, no matter what the cost was, both in dollars and in heartbreak. It would probably be far away, so we could expect to be separated for months at a time. It was the only thing left to do.

I investigated every public and private facility for boys in the country. Finally, I found a referral agency that specialized in placing children based on their individual histories and needs. The process was thorough and rigorous. I was given the name of a therapeutic, working ranch in the southern part of Utah—miles and miles from anywhere, which specializes in troubled youth, ages 9 to 14. The average length of treatment is 9 to 16 months. The estimation for Jeffrey's stay would be 16 to 24 months.

The High Top Ranch's philosophy is that kids are not like watches: they can't be fixed with a screwdriver. Instead, they teach new ways of living with an emphasis on ranching, farming, camping, and country living. Most of the staff is family and there is an emphasis on morality and family values. In a way, it's like stepping back in time when you're there—like generations before us, they work hard, play hard, and respect others. They love God, family, and community.

I carefully checked their references. Then Bob and I sat down with my parents. The decision was mine, but I needed everyone's support and agreement. To say that it was agonizing would do it no justice. I even consulted Scott's father, Jeffrey's paternal grandfather. "When you have but one choice, you have no choice," he said. We were sending him away—something we had fought against for years.

Jeffrey was accepted at High Top Ranch on August 23, 2003. He was to leave in two weeks, and he knew nothing about it. I knew his reaction would be explosive and that he would be very angry with us. Those two weeks were torture. My family and I agreed, though; it was time to be proactive, not reactive. With the doctors, we had tended to take a passive role. Though I'd resisted certain medications, and even refused some, I had usually given in to the doctors' "professional expertise." When we had ventured out on our own, we had found the only treatment that had ever been effective—medical marijuana. Our decision to send Jeff to the Ranch was reached with the same logic. If all the "system" could offer was a Level 14 public facility, or worse, we had to take the initiative to find him a more nurturing and secure environment.

Medical marijuana had given Jeffrey two years to grow and mature. It is impossible to know what path his therapy would have followed if his treatment had not been disrupted by federal government intervention. Instead we were forced to take another path. We only hoped the progress he'd made during those years would help him respond to the kind of therapy the Ranch offered.

While Jeffrey had no idea of our plan, we still had to do all the prep work to get everything ready. He needed clothes, boots, a bedspread—everything on the list the Ranch had provided. Every time I made a purchase and put it away, I cried. We decided that when the time came to tell him, we would tell him as a family. Jeff stayed with my parents for three days, and when they brought him home, we all sat down together. Bob gently explained that we all understood that he wasn't happy. Jeff actually agreed. I told him that there was a new school he was going to attend, not because he is bad, but because they had more people who could help him.

We weren't surprised when he blew up. Slowly, though, he began to deliberate about it. He realized and was able to admit that he really did want to get better. When he found out where the Ranch was, however, he went ballistic, yelling and slamming doors. He locked himself in the bathroom. We all knew that he was just as scared as he was mad.

I showed him pictures and told him about all of the animals and the beautiful fields and trees. Telling him on the eve of his departure left him little time to worry or act out over the decision, and he quickly resigned himself to the fact that he was going. His main concern was how long he would have to stay. He wondered if everybody would forget him. We all promised that we would write often, and that we would call and visit whenever his behavior allowed it. I cuddled with him the night before he left and we talked for a long time. He told me, "Mom, I want to be normal, I just don't know how."

❧

The next morning, August 23, 2003, we left early to reach the airport and fly to Utah. I was filled with mixed emotions after leaving him at the Ranch. I was so grateful that there was a safe place where he could potentially receive therapy, but I hurt so much in anticipation of our separation and his being so far away and so alone. The pain is still there for all of us, and we miss him desperately.

The staff there tells us that Jeff is one of their most difficult children, yet they adore him. One doctor compared him to a Jack Russell Terrier—little, smart, and afraid of nothing! Treatment and therapy without medication is encouraged. Jeffrey takes no medicine at the Ranch with the aim of observing and responding to his baseline behavior. He continues to have problems with aggression and controlling his behavior but is making positive strides. Unlike the previous residential placements where misconduct meant consequences of a "quiet room" or time out, the boys here earn X's that are worked off by such things as shoveling horse manure. It IS a working ranch! Rewards for good behavior can be as simple as being pulled on an inner tube in the snow behind the ATV, or making an off-campus trip to the closest town with staff members to go bowling, eat out, or shop. It's a simple life. One night on the phone I asked Jeff if there was anything he needed. He said, "No, there's nothing I really need. But I would sure like to have some shampoo that smells good!"

This ranch has a different environment than any of the places Jeff has been before. The boys are encouraged to develop a humble and positive attitude. Jeffrey doesn't whine on the phone; he doesn't complain (except that he is homesick); and he is truly grateful when we send him something. I can't help but compare that to the Christmas we'd spent two years before. He seldom writes letters, but he loves to get mail. Apparently, Jeffrey gets more letters than anyone else there, and that makes him feel good.

Jeff tells me that he is working on his issues. He asked me if I still "love his guts" even though he hasn't been very good. I assured him that would never ever change. He is starting to recognize that his behavior is sometimes outlandish and that certain thoughts trigger his outbursts. His doors of perception are slowly opening.

There are many animals at the Ranch, and Jeffrey's abusive behavior has stopped completely. The first time a staff member took Jeff to see the horses, he insisted that he knew how to mount a horse already—no one had to tell him how. So they let him climb up and get in the saddle. He knew how to get up there all right— he was just facing the wrong direction. He didn't become enraged, though, or think that people were laughing at him this time—he even cracked himself up.

Even though Jeff isn't at home, we talk about him all the time, and we realize how many good times we had, too. When Jeffrey was seven, my mom started reading to him during bath time from the Hardy Boys series of books. He was mesmerized by the suspense, sometimes gasping as he tried to guess what would happen next. Now that he is away in Utah, she still keeps the book on the back of the toilet tank. She says it reminds her of all the fun times they had together—that we all had together—that we all will have together again someday.

Jeffrey was constantly faced with changes in his life. He was moved back and forth, he lost his father, he was ejected from a dozen schools, he lived in both psychiatric hospitals and residential placement centers—he had a life that would challenge anyone of any age. The one thing he could always count on—and will always be able to count on—is his mom, his grandma and grandpa, and his family. We will always be here. That is a promise never to be broken.

If Jeff is certain of one thing, it's that his family adores him and will go to any length to protect and help him. I know this trust will help him continue to change. He has a long way to go before he is done, but I believe he's on his way. With some admittedly difficult work ahead, the staff sees promise with continued therapy. We remain hopeful about Jeffrey's recovery and his future.

Endnote

I would encourage any family who has experienced similar problems with a child to "keep on keeping on." Never give up hope that something will help your child. If the medications that have been prescribed by your doctors don't work, or make your children more ill, don't be afraid to consider alternatives. Do research. Discuss the possibility of medical marijuana treatment with your doctor. It wasn't long ago that I was opposed, because I was uneducated. Educate yourself, and then educate your doctor.

We don't have any doubts about whether medical marijuana helped Jeffrey. Our experience validates the fact that marijuana is a complicated, misunderstood medication. Incredibly, despite the mounting evidence that marijuana has medicinal value, the battle for its legal use continues. It remains legal in the state of California, but illegal federally. This battle is, in many cases, being fought by the seriously ill and those who love them. When battles are lost, lives are literally at stake.

For more information, or if you would like to take a stand in this profoundly significant matter, please refer to the organizations noted in the back of this book. It is our hope that the story of our journey will serve to aid other people in need.

Appendix 1: Is It Ethical and Legal to Give a Child Medical Marijuana?

Peter A. Clark, SJ, PhD
John McShain Chair in Ethics
Saint Joseph's University
5600 City Avenue
Philadelphia, Pennsylvania 19131
pclark@sju.edu

Affiliated Scholar at the Center for Clinical Bioethics
Georgetown University
Washington, D.C.

Bioethicist
Mercy Health System
Philadelphia, Pennsylvania

The use of medical marijuana in Jeffrey's case has legal, ethical and medical implications for minors not only in California but nationwide. Namely, it confronts whether medical marijuana was legal, ethical and in this child's best interest.

California's Proposition 215--or the Compassionate Care Act of 1996—states that one purpose of this Act is: "to ensure that seriously ill Californians have the right to obtain and use marijuana for medical purposes where that medical use is deemed appropriate and has been recommended by a physician who has determined that the person's health would benefit from the use of marijuana in the treatment of cancer, anorexia, AIDS, chronic pain, spasticity, glaucoma, arthritis, migraine, or any other illness for which marijuana provides relief."

Jeffrey appears to meet the criteria of the Act because he is seriously ill, his pediatrician believes that marijuana is medically appropriate under the circumstances and he benefited from the treatment. The issue in this case is whether or not it is legal and ethical for a parent/surrogate to give consent for a minor to use medical marijuana, which the federal government maintains is unproven in terms of safety and efficacy and could be a "gateway drug" that leads to more serious drug use.

On March 17, 1999, the most comprehensive analysis to date of medical literature about marijuana was issued by a White House commissioned committee of eleven independent scientists appointed by the

Institute of Medicine (IOM). The report concluded that the benefits of smoking marijuana were limited by the toxic effects of the smoke, but nonetheless recommended that the drug be given under close supervision to patients who do not respond to other therapies. It also stated that there was no evidence that giving the drug to sick people would increase illicit drug use in the general population. Nor is marijuana a "gateway drug" that prompts patients to use harder drugs like cocaine and heroin. This report shows that the concerns of the federal government are clearly unfounded and the failure of the federal government to reclassify marijuana as a Schedule II drug is jeopardizing the health and safety of many Americans.

To deny physicians the right to prescribe a therapy that relieves pain and suffering is to violate the physician–patient relationship. Patients/ surrogates have the right to expect full disclosure of all possible treatment options from their physicians, so that they can make informed medical decisions regarding their health. Physicians have the medical responsibility to provide adequate relief from both pain and suffering in order to give their patients an acceptable quality of life.

Failure to offer an available therapy that has proven to be effective would violate the basic ethical principle of non-maleficence, which prohibits infliction of harm, injury, or death, and is related to the maxim primum non nocere ("above all, or first, do no harm"), which is widely used to describe the duties of physicians. To allow any patient to suffer needlessly when the suffering can be relieved, whether that patient is an adult or a child, is to do direct harm to the patient. Therefore, it is in the patient's best interest that they, or in the case of a minor, their parents or surrogates, have the right to request medical marijuana under certain circumstances and physicians have the duty to disclose medical marijuana as an option and prescribe it when appropriate.

Scientific data has shown that the benefits of medical marijuana far outweigh the burdens. However, there is a need for continued research both in regards to maximizing marijuana's therapeutic effects and minimizing its adverse effects. The failure of the federal government to expand its funding for research on the medical use of marijuana in order to assess its effectiveness and safety is not only an affront to medical research, but it is also an injustice because it negates the best interest of the common good.

Seriously ill patients, both adults and minors, have the right to effective therapies. To deny them access to such therapies is to deny them the dignity and respect all persons deserve. Jeffrey's mother acted in her child's best interest. The benefits of treatment outweighed the burdens. No other medication or therapy was as effective as the use of medical marijuana in relieving his pain and suffering.

Finally, Jeffrey's quality of life not only improved but allowed him to gain self-esteem, real happiness and peace of mind. Allowing Jeffrey to use medical marijuana is not only in his best interest but also promotes the greater good in spite of the potential evil consequences.

Appendix 2: Resources

Organizations

Americans for Safe Access (ASA)
1678 Shattuck Ave. #317
Berkeley, CA 94709
Phone: (510) 486-8083
Fax: (510) 486-8090
Email: info@safeaccessnow.org

Coalition for Medical Marijuana
CSDP - CA Project
3220 N Street NW #141
Washington, DC 20007
info@csdp.org
www.medicalmj.org

Drug Policy Alliance
(formerly the Lindesmith Center-Drug Policy Foundation)
www.drugpolicy.org

New York
70 West 36th Street
16th Floor
New York, NY 10018
Phone: (212) 613-8020
Fax: (212) 613-8021
nyc@drugpolicy.org

Washington, DC
925 15th Street NW
2nd Floor
Washington, DC 20005
Phone: (202) 216-0035
Fax: (202) 216-0803
dc@drugpolicy.org

Drug Policy Alliance (continued)

San Francisco
2233 Lombard St
San Francisco, CA 94123
Phone: (415) 921-4987
Fax: (415) 921-1912
sf@drugpolicy.org

New Jersey
119 South Warren Street, 1st Fl
Trenton, NJ 08608
Phone: (609) 396-8613
Fax: (609) 396-9478
nj@drugpolicy.org

New Mexico
1227 Paseo de Peralta
Santa Fe, NM 87501
Phone: (505) 983-3277
Fax: (505) 983-3278
nm@drugpolicy.org

Sacramento
1225 8th Street, Suite 570
Sacramento,CA 95814
Phone: (916) 444-3751
Fax: (916) 444-3802
sacto@drugpolicy.org

Legal Affairs
717 Washington Street
Oakland, CA 94607
Phone: (510) 208-7711
Fax: (510) 208-7722
legalaffairs@drugpolicy.org

Green Aid
84 Lake Park Ave. #172
Oakland, CA 94610
1-888-271-7674
info@green-aid.com

Marijuana Policy Project (MPP)
PO Box 77492
Capitol Hill
Washington, DC 20013
(202)-462-5747
info@mpp.org
www.mpp.org

NORML (National Organization for the Reform of Marijuana Laws)
1600 K Street, NW
Suite 501
Washington, DC 20006-2832
Phone: (202) 483-5500
Fax: (202) 483-0057
norml@norml.org
www.norml.org

NORML, California Chapter
San Francisco Office
2215-R Market St. #278
San Francisco, CA 94114
San Francisco: (415) 563-5858
East Bay: (510) 540-1066
Fax: (510) 849-3974
www.canorml.org

Los Angeles Office
8749 Holloway Dr.
W. Hollywood 90069
(310) 652-8654

Wo/Men's Alliance for Medical Marijuana (WAMM)
309 Cedar St. #39
Santa Cruz, California 95060.
Note: This is not WAMM's physical location.
(831) 423-5413
info@wamm.org
www.wamm.org

Appendix 3: References

In my initial research, I came across several very informative sites and books. I have listed a few of my favorites here. There is a host of information at the library, bookstores and on the Internet.

Websites

www.wamm.org
www.norml.org
www.drugpolicy.org
www.rxmarijuana.com (Hosted by **Lester Grinspoon, MD**, Professor of Psychiatry Emeritus at the Harvard Medical School and **James Bakalar, J.D.**, Lecturer in Law in the Department of Psychiatry at the Harvard Medical School.)

Books

Dr. Lester Grinspoon, *Marihuana Reconsidered.* Harvard University Press, 1971, revised 1977.
Dr. Lester Grinspoon and James Bakalar, *Marihuana, the Forbidden Medicine.* Yale University Press, 1997.
Leslie L.Iverson, *The Science of Marijuana.* Oxford University Press, 2000.
Physicians' Desk Reference (PDR). Medical Economics Company, Montvale, New Jersey, 2001.